# The Simulated Patient Handbook

A COMPREHENSIVE GUIDE FOR FACILITATORS
AND SIMULATED PATIENTS

## FIONA DUDLEY

*Lecturer, facilitator, trainer and simulated patient*

Foreword by

## JONATHAN SILVERMAN

*Associate Clinical Dean and Director of Communication Studies*
*School of Clinical Medicine*
*University of Cambridge*

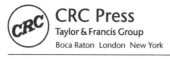

CRC Press
Taylor & Francis Group
Boca Raton London New York

CRC Press is an imprint of the
Taylor & Francis Group, an **informa** business

First published 2012 by Radcliffe Publishing

Published 2019 by CRC Press
Taylor & Francis Group
6000 Broken Sound Parkway NW, Suite 300
Boca Raton, FL 33487-2742

ISBN-13: 978-1-84619-454-2 (pbk)

**Visit the Taylor & Francis Web site at
http://www.taylorandfrancis.com**

**and the CRC Press Web site at
http://www.crcpress.com**

Fiona Dudley has asserted her right under the Copyright, Designs and Patents Act 1988 to be identified as the author of this work.

British Library Cataloguing in Publication Data

A catalogue record for this book is available from the British Library.

Typeset by Darkriver Design, Auckland, New Zealand

# Contents

# Foreword

The exponential rise in the adoption of simulated patients into mainstream medical education has been truly phenomenal. Who would have predicted 20 years ago that medical undergraduate finals examinations would regularly feature simulated rather than real patients? Who would have thought that post-graduate qualifications such as the MRCP, FRCA and the MRCGP would adopt the use of simulated patients as an established component of their examination processes? And who would have even considered that working with simulated patients to practice interviewing skills would not just be commonplace but an extensive, established, mandatory feature of medical education in most if not all medical schools in the United Kingdom? Eighteen years ago, I started to think about how to establish a team of simulated patients to use in medical education in the East of England. We began working with two regular actors. Our medical school now employs a simulated patient director and we have over 130 simulated patients servicing our undergraduate programme.

I always ask our new medical students why on earth we spend so much money and so much effort in training simulated patients when we have a hospital and community full of real patients who are only too willing to be interviewed by medical students. It does not take them long to realise what we can offer in our programme. Simulated patients provide a situation in which students can experiment and learn in a safe environment, without the possibility of harming real patients, yet in as close an approximation to reality as possible. Simulated patients provide ideal opportunities for rehearsal. Here is the ultimate offer to learners: feel free to experiment and to rehearse skills over and over again – do what you can rarely do with real patients in the outside world, say out loud 'that didn't seem to work very well, let me try it again differently'. Simulated patients are willing for learners to make mistakes and to provide multiple opportunities for trial and error so that learners can practice skills in safety without any adverse consequences of 'botching' an attempt at a new skill. Just think about the impossibility of using real patients to teach learners about interviewing an angry patient who has been kept waiting for a long time, or giving the diagnosis of multiple sclerosis to somebody and breaking that bad news for the first time, or talking to the parent of a child who has just been killed in a road traffic accident. Yet in the simulated situation, learners can obtain feedback from peers, patient and facilitator and learn behaviours which will enable them to be much more effective and supportive when later on, in real-life, they face similar difficult and challenging issues.

Communication skills teaching relies heavily on experiential methodology utilising active learning in small groups, video recordings, simulated patients and constructive feedback. In recent years, considerable effort has been employed in training facilitators to teach communication skills effectively using these approaches. And of course, it is now being realised that simulated patients need considerable training and help too. Their increasing numbers has now led to efforts to professionalise simulated patient training. Simulated patients trainers in undergraduate medical schools in the UK have come together through the SPOTS organisation and have held regular national meetings. And a national meeting of medical educators has looked specifically at the use of non-clinical teachers in medical education and at ways in which standards could be set and training maximised.

However, there has been little in the way of handbooks concerning specifically the use of simulated patients and much training has been by word of mouth. Fortunately this excellent manual goes some way to redressing this deficiency. Fiona has extensive experience as both a simulated patient and a facilitator and she has clearly written this handbook from the heart. She has brought together all her experience in a highly accessible way that addresses the needs of all those working as a simulated patient or with simulated patients. Simulated patients will find this book collates so many good tips and advice about how to work with learners. Facilitators working with simulated patients will read this book in order to get a clearer insight into what simulated patients need from them and how to work together as an effective team.

This book clearly describes the variety of backgrounds, not necessarily acting, from which simulated patients can be drawn and the need for recruitment from all aspects of society in order to mirror the patients that learners will meet in real-life. It covers the attributes required to work effectively in this field. What stands out most strongly here is the author's keen appreciation of the need for anyone working in this way to be on the side of the learner, to be there to help them rather than hinder them and to appreciate what a difficult and important job it is to be a health professional.

The manual covers different approaches that can be taken to the use of simulated patients, the ways in which simulated patients are used in both formative teaching and summative examinations and is particularly strong about how to give feedback, both in role, out of role and in neutral. It also covers just how closely a simulated patient has to work with the facilitator and the need for discussion both before and after teaching sessions in order to maximise potential benefits.

Communication skills teaching in medicine has now come of age. Many of the battles have been won and communication skills teaching and assessment have become established as central core components of the medical education landscape. What is needed now is dissemination of good practice and practical thoughtful help to turn good intentions into excellent teaching and evaluation. Fiona Dudley's book provides this help and I would highly commend it to all simulated patients and facilitators

Jonathan Silverman
Associate Clinical Dean and Director of Communication Studies
School of Clinical Medicine
University of Cambridge
*October 2011*

# About the author

After completing a Russian degree and spending a few years travelling, Fiona returned to England to train as an occupational therapist. She worked for several years in the fields of adult and child mental health until deciding to become a full-time mum. She began to work as a simulated patient in the early days of their development in this country. During the last 20 years she has worked increasingly and extensively in the field of medical and healthcare education as a lecturer, facilitator, trainer and, of course, simulated patient. She has worked for a variety of institutions, including the Leeds School of Medicine; the Hull and York Medical School, the Yorkshire and the Humber Strategic Health Authority; the Yorkshire Deanery; and Peninsula Medical School. She is also an active member of the Simulated Patient Organisers and Trainers organisation, which continues to share best practice and develop the creative use of simulated patients nationwide. This book is the culmination of her experiences of all aspects of working with simulated patients.

# Acknowledgements

This book has been a while in the making and so many lovely friends and colleagues have helped and inspired me along the way that it would be impossible to mention all by name.

Some have given specific help and guidance with the writing, so thanks to Steve Attmore, Dean Brown, Steve Duffy, Miriam Hawkins and Jonathan Silverman.

Thanks also to my dear friends from the simulated patient community for all their support, encouragement and friendship (not to mention the laughs!) over the past twenty years, especially Ian Baxter, Kieran Conlan, Jenny Dent, Jem Dobbs, Alison George, Nabeela Azhar Ibrahim, Alf Israel, Tracey Lucas, Tony Martin, Hayley Mason, Martina McClements, Robina Mir, Belinda Noda, Cassie Reynolds, Cynthia Rover, Maggi Stratford, Narelle Summers, Val Tagger, Godfrey Thorpe, Chris Thomas, Tony Walford, Jane Whittaker, Sally Womersley and Andy Worthington.

Thanks to my many friends and colleagues at Hull York Medical School – especially Andy Brown, Sarah Collins, Jay Exley, Anna Hammond and Lesley Jones.

Many thanks also to Iain Wilkinson and Alison Kitch from the Strategic Health Authority, and to the rest of the training team there – Kate Barker, Daphne Franks and Alistair Imrie.

Thanks also to friends and colleagues, past and present, at Leeds Medical School – Alison Ashworth, Len Biran, Adrian Boonin, Barbara Dransfield, Sarah Escott, Anne-Marie Howes, Rob Lane, Olwyn Marshall, Penny Morris, Gail Nicholls, Bernard and Kay Pierce, Miranda Powers, Emma Storr, Jools Symmons, Ann Wilcock.

Thanks to Karen Roberts and Ramesh Mehay at the Yorkshire Deanery, and Rob Johnson at Peninsula Medical School.

I am also grateful for the enthusiasm of members of the Simulated Patient Organisers and Trainers organisation . . . especially Karen Barry, Frank Coffey, Libby Dicken, Michelle Gutteridge, Carrie Hamilton, Pene Herman Smith, Byron McGuiness, Alison Whitfield.

Many thanks also for the wisdom and expertise of Jamie Etherington and Gillian Nineham at Radcliffe Publishing Ltd, and Camille Lowe at Undercover project management.

And to all the other wonderful simulated patients, academic staff, facilitators and administration bods who have made this field such a fun and exciting one in which to work.

This book is dedicated to the cherished
memory of my mum and dad, and to the
precious inspiration of my lovely children,
Kiera, Seth and Luka – thank you!

# PART ONE

# Background

*I hear and I forget.*
*I see and I remember.*
*I do and I understand.*

Confucius (551–479 BC)

# CHAPTER 1

# So you want to join the world of the simulated patient?

There can be no such thing as 'The Definitive Guide' to working as or with a simulated patient. There are so many potential situations you may encounter, so many variations of ways in which you can work, that it would be impossible to cover every aspect of the work in one small tome. This handbook is intended to give you an insight into the world of consultation skills training using simulated patients, from all perspectives, and to give facilitators and simulators alike some guidelines and practical advice about how best to manage such opportunities. It provides useful information and ideas for further development of your own skills and it should inspire you to continue to explore the creative potential of working with simulated patients.

Assuming that you chose this book with a particular aim in mind, rather than just randomly selecting it from the bookshelf for a good bedtime read (it could be a bit thin on the plot line!), you probably have some idea of what simulated patients are and what they can do. However, opinions are usually formed from experience, and so if you have only encountered simulated patients in limited settings such as examination situations or undergraduate medical education sessions, you could be surprised at the versatility of simulated patients as a resource. Therefore, for the sake of clarity, I will attempt a brief definition that will be expanded throughout the book as we explore the different areas of potential work with simulated patients.

## WHAT EXACTLY IS A SIMULATED PATIENT?

A simulated patient is a person who pretends to be a patient (or, indeed, as we shall see, a relative or even a health practitioner), simulating health problems in order to offer health professionals an opportunity to develop, practise and be assessed on their consultation skills and providing feedback.

A simulated patient is an *ordinary* person (the green antennae only develop with experience!). The simulated patient may be young or old, fat or thin, tall or short, black, white or grey. They may have no drama training whatsoever or they may be a trained actor. They may have some medical knowledge or none at all.

They may have qualifications coming out of their ears or they may have left school after 11 years of playing hookey.

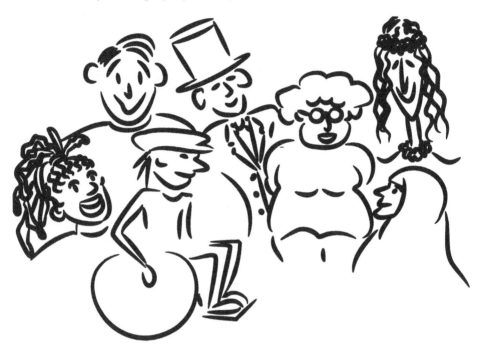

**Potential simulated patients**

Basically, whatever a person's physical or psychological attributes, whatever their educational or professional experience, they have the potential to work as a simulated patient. Because patients are drawn from a whole cross-section of society, this diversity needs to be reflected in the variety of people working as simulated patients.

To say that everybody has the potential to become a simulated patient is not, however, to say that everybody has the potential to be an effective simulated patient. There are certain personal attributes that are essential, and others that are highly desirable, for the people to have who wish to carry out this work. Some of these are innate personal qualities; others may be acquired and developed through training and experience.

Simulated patients are asked to do many different kinds of work, from examinations for medical students to interviews for practice managers in surgeries, from 'mystery shopper' customer service training for pharmacists to breaking bad news for people working in hospices. The ways in which simulated patients may be used are limited only by the imagination. Each different way of working requires certain particular qualities from the simulated patient, as we shall soon see.

## AND WHAT DO YOU DO WITH ONE?

The use of simulated interactions as a method of teaching consultation skills has gained immensely in popularity over the last few years. As a consequence, it happens increasingly that people who have little or no experience of working with simulated patients in their teaching are finding themselves in the exciting, if somewhat daunting, position of facilitating a simulated patient session.

It may be that you are a clinician who has been asked to carry out some consultation skills training with your colleagues. Perhaps you work in higher education with healthcare students and need to facilitate one of the increasing number of communication sessions within the modern curriculum. It may be that you have worked as a simulated patient but never in the role of facilitator. Whatever the reason, you should realise that this is no ordinary teaching session and the effective facilitation of the simulated patient session requires no ordinary teaching skills!

Teaching using simulated patients is not so much an imparting of knowledge as an exploration, by a group of people, of a particular given situation, in the hope that the most effective strategies of dealing with the challenges presented will emerge. Therefore, teaching using simulated patients may require a different approach and attitude for those accustomed to a more didactic style of teaching. Generally speaking, as a teacher, you are usually able to thoroughly prepare the material you wish to present to the students – you can even practise the way in which you wish to present it. In the simulated patient session, you can prepare and practise your introduction, but beyond that you must be completely responsive to the situation and draw your teaching material from the interactions presented.

Although each consultation will have its own learning objectives, which the scenarios will have been developed to present, it is a wholly interactive teaching method. Neither the facilitator nor the participants can ever know exactly what will arise during the course of the session. It is vital, therefore, that you are flexible and creative enough to react to any given situation and that you are able to draw the learning points from what does arise, in a spontaneous fashion. Now, before you panic and decide to apply for a job at your local supermarket instead, try to consider the opportunity to work in this way as a unique and exciting challenge! With a little preparation and careful thought, and a lot of enthusiasm, you should find working with simulated patients a most fulfilling and rewarding exercise.

In this handbook, I will endeavour to give you some guidelines and direction, some advice and some top tips, to help you feel confident in approaching this challenge and ensure you get the most benefit from the session, for your group of practitioners and for yourself. There are, as in all aspects of work with simulated patients, no hard and fast rules. As I have mentioned, there are so many different ways simulated patients can be used in the teaching and assessment of consultation skills, it is impossible to give definitive approaches to any of the work. However, in this handbook I have aimed to give you as comprehensive a guide as possible to various potential ways of working with simulated patients, focusing in detail on the most common techniques and approaches. It is important that as you read this, perhaps with a view to running a session, you bear in mind the learning outcomes you are hoping to achieve and the nature of the group of people with whom you are working. Ideas and guidance are offered here to help you decide what will work best for you and your group, and to help you develop your own style and techniques, according to your own personality and experience. Explore and create!

## WHERE ARE YOU FROM?

> *The art of teaching is*
> *the art of assisting discovery.*
>
> Mark Van Doren (1894–1972)

People from many different backgrounds can facilitate simulated patient sessions. Your own background and experience will make a difference to the type of sessions you can most effectively facilitate, as well as obviously making a difference to how you run those sessions. There are no absolute dictates about this, as each session will be a unique venture. However, it is important that you are able to reflect honestly on yourself and your skills, to ensure that you have the relevant qualifications, experience and even personality to be effective in this role, before embarking on this challenge.

If you are a simulated patient from a drama background, for example, you may be very good at facilitating a forum session on managing conflict between professionals. However, the clinical support you would need to enable you to facilitate a management planning session for complex medical consultations, for example, may make the situation too challenging and therefore ineffective as a learning medium for practitioners. Equally, a palliative care consultant may be very skilled at facilitating a session on breaking bad news for medical students, but may find a forum session for receptionists on dealing with angry patients rather more challenging.

Therefore, before accepting the challenge of facilitation, it is important that you are very clear about the learning objectives of the session and the experience level of the group you are working with. Make an honest appraisal of your own capabilities and, if possible, only agree to facilitate those sessions that you feel confident of managing effectively.

If you are used to more didactic teaching methods, working with simulated patients can be a precarious experience. As an experienced teacher, even though you may be very clear about how different the job of facilitating a simulated patient session is, you may find it all too easy to slip back into the 'imparting of information' model. It may be more comfortable for you to pass on your own knowledge and experience to a group, but it is essential that you are awake to this process throughout the session. Your job is to facilitate their learning experience, not to 'teach' them how to do it. You should be encouraging each practitioner to analyse his or her own strengths and weaknesses. They can do this with the help and support of their colleagues within the group, and their analysis should be backed up, or disputed, by the simulated patient. You, as facilitator, can then further reinforce aspects of the consultations and identify any learning points that might have been missed in discussion. By encouraging them to work together to explore different options and to find their own solutions, you will be a more effective educator than if you continually give them your own opinions. This is not to say that you should not share some of your own experience and knowledge with the group; however, the more involved they can be in their own learning process, the more robust the learning will be.

## JARGON BUSTER AND GLOSSARY OF TERMS

> *Think like a wise man*
> *but communicate in the*
> *language of the people.*
> William Butler Yeats (1865–1939)

One aspect of consultation skills that is often highlighted during training sessions involving simulated patients is the use of jargon. For clarity's sake I will define here the basic terms I have used in this book. A more comprehensive and alphabetised 'jargon buster' can be found in Appendix 1.

**Simulated patient** – I hope you will be aware of what a simulated patient is by the time you have read this handbook . . . but you should be aware that they may also be called an SP, a role player, a patient teacher, a simulator, an actor, a standardised patient, a character, a patient, a co-facilitator, a programmed patient, a clinical teaching associate, a co-teacher . . . and probably a host of other names we shan't go into here! I have used the terms 'simulated patient' and 'simulator' when talking about teaching sessions and the term 'standardised patient' when describing the simulated patient in an assessment situation.

**Facilitator** – the facilitator is the person who is coordinating the session. They are responsible for guiding the simulated patient and the group of learners in order to bring out learning points relevant to the aims of the session. The facilitator may have a completely different role outside the session (e.g. doctor, teacher, nurse, service user, or they may be from any number of other professions or have any number of other experiences). Although their role outside the session will obviously influence the way it is conducted, within the session they are there primarily to facilitate the learning of the group members.

**Feedback** – this is the means by which the simulated patient, the facilitator and the other group members help the practitioner to see and understand their own strengths, and to identify the areas where they may wish to improve their skills by practising different approaches and developing new ideas. There are two sections in this book that cover some of the different ways in which feedback can be given, both in the feedback you can expect from the simulated patient and in the feedback you can encourage your group members to give.

**Practitioner** – there are so many different health professionals at so many levels of training who now work with simulated patients, I have chosen the generic term 'practitioner' to describe them, whether they be receptionist, midwife, domestic or social worker, student, consultant or volunteer.

**Training provider** – this is the term I have chosen to use to describe the person or organisation that employs simulated patients and facilitators for any given work. It also refers, in this instance, to appraising or organising bodies in the case of examinations or interviews.

**In role/out of role/role neutral** – this describes the ways in which a simulated patient can be participating in different parts of the session. **In role** is the part of the session when the simulated patient is playing the role of the character, whether within the consultation or during feedback. **Out of role** is the part of the session when the simulated patient speaks as himself/herself. **Role neutral** is sometimes used to describe any parts of the session when the simulated patient is required to remain in role but outside the immediate situation and emotion of the consultation. This may be useful if the group wishes to 'hot-seat' the patient (a process described later in the book), or if you would like them to give feedback in role but without the heightened emotions that may have been displayed during the consultation itself.

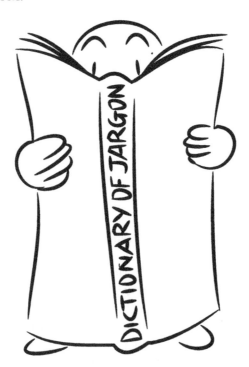

'It must have "hieroglyphic globalotomy" in here somewhere . . !'

# CHAPTER 2

# Consultation skills training: how important is it?

*Communication is a core clinical skill: it is not simply*
*being nice to patients or being patient centred*
*but an essential component that determines*
*our clinical effectiveness.*

Jonathan Silverman

In order to become an effective facilitator and for the success of the session, it is absolutely vital that you believe in what you are doing. This may sound ridiculously self-evident, but it seems that sometimes people who have clearly failed to appreciate the importance of such training for health professionals can find themselves in the position of facilitating simulated patient sessions! Hoping that you do not fall into this category, but recognising that you may, I will briefly outline the benefits of consultation skills training in general and consultation skills training using simulated patients.

## CONSULTATION SKILLS TRAINING IN GENERAL

Increasingly the benefits of effective consultation skills are being researched and acknowledged. However, as with everything in times of economic constraint, effective consultation skills sometimes need defending when held in comparison with more measurable skills. There has now been plenty of research showing the advantages of mandatory training in the specifics of managing a consultation, as well as in interpersonal communication with patients, relatives and colleagues in general. The benefits derived from consultation skills training can be divided into two broad categories: patient well-being and efficiency. Inevitably, happier patients and more effective management techniques can only lead to improved job satisfaction for practitioners.

**Patient well-being**
➤ Patients are happier and more willing to consult with a practitioner who shows respect and empathy.
➤ An improvement in the relationship between patient and practitioner leads to more open communication.
➤ An effective consultation will improve patient understanding, thus giving the patient greater autonomy and control over their own treatment options.
➤ A patient who is satisfied with a consultation will develop more confidence in the practitioner and is therefore more likely to engage in a treatment programme promoted by that practitioner. Currently, a large percentage of prescriptions are not collected from the pharmacist, often because a patient is not confident that the practitioner has understood their problem and offered appropriate treatment.

**Efficiency and cost-effectiveness**
➤ Although it may seem to take longer and therefore cost more to conduct a patient-centred consultation, the fact that it leads to a more thorough gathering of information and consequently to more accurate diagnoses makes the long-term effects more cost-effective.
➤ An improved relationship and better communication between practitioner and patient may lead to more accurate diagnoses sooner. For example, where a patient may repeatedly attend with a variety of complaints, a skilfully managed consultation may discover the underlying cause far earlier, thus saving time and resources in the longer term.
➤ By exploring different methods of dealing with potentially difficult consultations, the practitioner can learn to better manage challenging situations and may be more likely to achieve a positive outcome to the consultation.
➤ The practitioner can improve their time-management skills by learning how to structure consultations.
➤ Practitioners will often be offered training for specific situations or tasks. These include breaking bad news, dealing with aggressive patients, managing challenging consultations, dealing with drug users, managing staff conflict and so forth. Ultimately, all of these done well will improve patient and practitioner well-being and will increase satisfaction, efficiency and cost-effectiveness.
➤ Practitioners are often required to undergo training to help them communicate better with colleagues and fellow professionals. They may then be required to demonstrate their skills in communication, in appraisal situations or in practising different ways of dealing with incidences of conflict between professionals. Improved communication between professionals results in better teamwork and, ultimately, better care for the patients.

Simulated patients are also used in situations where a doctor or other healthcare professional has got into legal difficulties and needs some extra training on their communication skills as part of the remedial measures suggested.

Having accepted the necessity of consultation skills training in principle, let us now consider the advantages of working with simulated patients as a methodology.

## SO WHY CHOOSE TO WORK WITH SIMULATED PATIENTS?

So why would you choose this way of teaching, which is in so many ways more challenging and is often more expensive than other forms of training in consultation skills? Simulated patients were first used in the training of medical students in 1963. An American neurologist, Howard S Barrows, introduced trained actors to play the roles of patients, to provide an opportunity for the medical students he was teaching to practise their clinical skills. He saw the value and potential

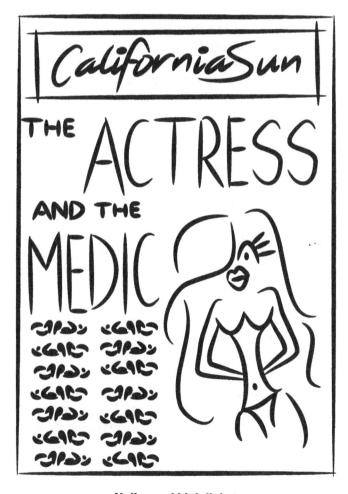

**Hollywood high jinks!**

of using them as standardised or simulated patients in both the evaluation and, later, in the teaching of medical students. Although he was a respected clinician and educator, Barrows was heavily criticised by colleagues who felt that by doing this he was damaging their profession. Despite sensationalist newspaper headlines, he continued to promote the use of simulated patients and experiential education, as he firmly believed that students should learn in the same ways that they will practise. Flight simulation as a way of training pilots had been accepted since the inception of manned flight. Barrows therefore felt it was equally valid to use a simulated patient for the training of doctors.

Working with simulated patients has grown hugely since those early days, as a way of developing the skills of health practitioners in dealing with patients, relatives and one another. There are many different ways of cultivating these skills, but the use of simulated patients can definitely reach parts that other methods cannot.

Of course there is much to be learnt from didactic lectures or paper/web-based learning. Of course there are other interactive ways of exploring consultation skills issues and analysing and practising skills. However, because working with simulated patients is so interactive and engaging, it can provide a learning experience that is at once both broader and deeper. It can also provide material to suit different learning styles, which is then processed on different levels – on an emotional level, on an intellectual level and on a contextual level.

If we look briefly at the ways in which consultation skills can be learnt and practised, we see that each has its advantages and its disadvantages. Even though working with simulated patients also has its drawbacks, we can see here that it often compensates for the failings of some of the other methods. Ideally, a variety of methods should be employed to gain maximum benefit.

➤ Practitioners can watch and analyse consultations performed by others. This can be through watching 'live' consultations in practice or by watching recordings. This can be valuable in learning to identify certain skills and witness their potential effects. However, this method gives no indication as to the practitioner's own capabilities and it offers no guidance as to where they could improve and how.

➤ Practitioners can record their own actual consultations. There is a great deal of value in this practice if it is logistically viable. However, they will only be able to use those recordings from consultations that were consented to by the patients, leaving perhaps the more challenging consultations unrecorded. Also, although the recording can be analysed afterwards, there is no opportunity to find out how the behaviours and words of the practitioner actually impacted on the patient. Equally, it gives no chance for the practitioner to explore other strategies or to try out other techniques.

➤ Healthcare professionals and students can be observed practising carrying out a consultation or part of a consultation by a clinician and then they can be given feedback about it. This presupposes a level of expertise (highly desirable before they are let loose on real patients!) and, again, is unlikely to give experience in the more challenging consultations. Using a simulated patient gives the opportunity for practice in a safe environment, whereby the practitioner can make mistakes in the secure knowledge that no patient will be affected. Also, as for practitioners recording their own actual consultations, alternative strategies cannot be explored and practised.

➤ Groups of practitioners can role-play various situations and practise their skills on one another. This can be very useful in many situations but it is often difficult to achieve in reality, as practitioners share a common level of knowledge. This can mean that they are often unable to realistically portray a patient, with the different level of knowledge and experience that person may have. A simulated patient will not have the same degree of professional knowledge and should, therefore, be able to give more natural responses within a consultation. 'Acting' with colleagues presents its own inherent challenges. Embarrassment is reduced by using simulated patients because, even though the practitioners know that they are not real patients, they are still 'real strangers', which adds an essential degree of realism to the situation. Simulated patients are also trained to portray a variety of roles effectively, which may be more difficult when performing 'in-house' role play. They are also trained to present the information in a useful way, offering it in chunks, in response to the skills demonstrated by the practitioner. If colleagues are role-playing with each other, they are often so preoccupied with 'acting the role' that they are unable to concentrate on the interviewing practitioner's skills. There may also be problems in ensuring sensitive and helpful feedback, since the atmosphere often created when practitioners are practising role play scenarios is often less conducive to thoughtful comments. There may be a tendency to give overcritical or bland, unconstructive feedback.

# PART TWO

# Preparation

*If I had six hours to chop down a tree,*
*I'd spend the first hour sharpening the axe.*
Abraham Lincoln (1809–1865)

# CHAPTER 3

# Recruiting simulated patients

Having decided that the most effective way to provide your consultation skills training is by using simulated patients, your next challenge is where to find them. This may not be your responsibility, as the organisation you are working with may have an established bank of simulated patients. However, if the task does fall to you, you should consider two options: using an agency or recruiting independently. There are clear advantages and disadvantages to each choice.

## USING AN AGENCY
### Advantages
➤ An agency has a wider pool of people on which to draw and therefore may be better able to provide suitable simulated patients.
➤ The simulated patients have usually received thorough training, and may even benefit from an appraisal scheme.
➤ If you explain to the agency what the learning objectives of your session/s are, they will often be able to provide suitable scenarios to help meet these.
➤ An agency will do all the administration for you, which can be a hidden cost and an onerous chore.
➤ If you are not happy with the work of an individual simulated patient, it is easier to complain to an agency, as it is less personal.

### Disadvantages
➤ An agency is usually more expensive, although it is important to be aware of the less obvious costs (e.g. administration), if deciding to recruit independently.
➤ Your communication with the simulated patient is usually less direct.
➤ You need to trust that the agency has understood your requirements and will provide an appropriate simulated patient.
➤ Sometimes the training the simulated patients have received is not completely in accordance with the way in which you would like them to work.
➤ There is more room for logistical difficulties as the process is less direct.

## RECRUITING INDEPENDENTLY

If you decide to recruit independently, it will remove the disadvantages as listed for when using an agency, but you will also, obviously, lose the advantages listed. Therefore, recruiting independently will demand greater organisational and creative input on your part.

You may decide to do the recruitment yourself, either for a one-off session or in order to build a bank of simulated patients for use in your own institution. Whatever your aims, you should consider the following points.

You need to find the people in the first place. These may be people you know or have heard of through friends. I have even recruited on trains and at bus stops (following ad hoc conversations, I hasten to add – I draw the line at stalking!), but there are plenty of more orthodox routes to take:

➤ contact healthcare institutions that already use simulated patients
➤ ask colleagues who have worked with simulated patients for recommendations
➤ if you participate in a consultation skills session yourself, ask for contact details from those simulated patients who impress you
➤ ask simulated patients for recommendations of colleagues
➤ approach educational institutions such as drama colleges who may or may not have experience of the work
➤ contact service user and community groups (this is especially useful if you are recruiting for a specialist group, e.g. bilingual simulated patients)
➤ approach amateur dramatic organisations
➤ look on the Internet for freelance simulated patients
➤ advertise in the local media.

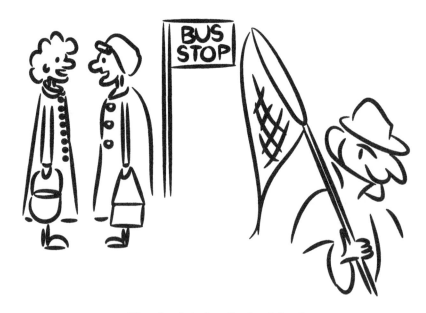

**The simulated patient catcher!**

Once you have recruited suitable people, you will need to train them. The amount of training and guidance the simulated patients will need depends very much on their background. A young actor, fresh out of drama school, will need a different kind of training from a person recruited from a community group, for example. This will be covered in more detail later in Chapter 4.

You will need to write scenarios for the session. You may choose to do so if you decide to use an agency, but if you are recruiting independently and therefore responsible for the whole process, you will have no choice but to do so. This is looked at in more depth in Chapter 5.

You will be responsible for all the administration for the session. This includes:

➤ making sure the simulated patients, facilitators and practitioners have all the necessary paperwork about the scenario
➤ making sure all parties have full logistical details such as the time and date of the session and directions to the venue
➤ making sure payment and expenses have been organised and details of rates of pay and methods of claiming have been communicated to the simulated patients and facilitators, and to the practitioners if they are able to claim any expenses
➤ devising, preparing, distributing and interpreting the feedback forms, should any evaluation of the session be required.

You will be responsible for the travel expenses of the simulators. If you are booking a group of simulated patients, it is worth considering their travel expenses and perhaps circulating contact details (having gained their consent for this) in the hope that they will be able to travel together and thus minimise the costs.

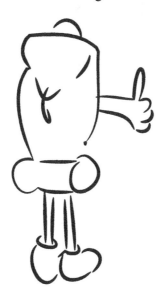

**Hitching a lift**

If such a decision lies with you, you will also need to decide how much to pay your simulated patients. Until a recognised accredited qualification and professional structure is developed, payment is very much dependent on the individual training provider. There is a vast range of levels of remuneration given to simulated patients, and much regional difference. Some simulated patients receive a sizeable fee for their services; others must content themselves with travel expenses and some tasty buns in the morning break! You could check with other local institutions to find out how much they are paying their role players, as if you offer significantly less, you will find it more difficult to recruit. When working out levels of remuneration, you should also consider what you are expecting them to do. Are you going to pay the same amount for a brief cameo appearance as for a 4-hour objective structured clinical examination? Are you going to pay the same amount for the portrayal of simple indigestion symptoms as for that of intense distress following the breaking of bad news? You should also bear in mind that many simulated patients are self-employed, and so, even if you only employ someone for an hour, it means that they would not be able to take any other work for that morning/afternoon/evening. I give you no answers, but simply urge you to be thoughtful about the decisions you make.

**Tax-free income**

# CHAPTER 4

# Training simulated patients

If you use an agency to provide your simulated patients, it is worth checking with the agency what level of training they have received, as this can vary considerably. You could reasonably expect that they have been trained to develop a basic role and to give constructive feedback. However, there are so many different ways simulated patients may be used, and therefore so many different ways they may be experienced in working, that it is important to match your own specific requirements with the experience and level of training of the simulated patient. You should be very clear as to your expectations of the simulated patient, therefore, when booking through an agency.

## CORE COMPETENCIES
Here is a breakdown of the skills you should expect your simulated patient to have, in order to provide an effective learning environment in a variety of situations.

### Basic core competencies for all sessions
All sessions require a simulated patient who is able to:
➤ develop and improvise a role
➤ learn crucial facts within the given scenario
➤ recall information in an appropriate way
➤ give sensitive, constructive feedback
➤ adapt easily to ever-changing requirements within the session
➤ understand the position of the simulated patient within the teaching situation
➤ work effectively as a team with the facilitator.

### Additional competencies essential for other areas
Examinations and recruitment interviews require a simulated patient who is able to:
➤ accurately recall learnt facts
➤ remain consistent in the role they portray
➤ chunk the information that they give appropriately

➤ make an objective assessment of a candidate's performance (if required)
➤ moderate a role to achieve consistency with other simulated patients playing the same role.

Forum theatre and cameo sessions require a simulated patient who is able to:
➤ learn a script
➤ take direction
➤ remain in role for extended periods
➤ respond directly to large groups of people.

Simulators simulating health professionals must be able to:
➤ assimilate appropriate professional attitude
➤ learn professional jargon.

Third-party consultations require simulated patients who can:
➤ comfortably respond to cues from another simulated patient
➤ demonstrate appropriate aspects of a relationship.

Bilingual scenarios require simulated patients who are able to:
➤ speak English and at least one other language fluently
➤ have an understanding of relevant cultural issues.

Practitioner-directed sessions require simulated patients who are able to:
➤ very quickly create a character
➤ analyse information to identify learning points
➤ improvise to a high level of expertise.

Self-facilitation requires highly skilled simulated patients who also have:
➤ facilitation skills
➤ organisational skills, to be clear of their role at all times during the session.

Simulating physical signs requires simulated patients who are able to:
➤ interpret and accurately portray a variety of signs to enable accurate diagnosis, based on physical examination.

When you are involved in training, assessing and monitoring the simulated patients, it is worth recording which sessions each simulated patient is suitable to undertake. For example, is this simulated patient:
➤ suitable for simple examination stations?
➤ suitable for complex examination stations?
➤ suitable for simple roles where feedback is required?
➤ suitable for complex roles where feedback is required?

Obviously, simulated patients will develop competencies to different standards. The more accurate your picture of their skills and strengths is, the more effectively you will be able to cast them in teaching sessions. For example, you may have a bilingual simulated patient who is brilliant at giving feedback but is less confident in acting a role. In a scenario focusing on the challenges of using an untrained interpreter, they could potentially play the patient, as they may only be required to describe their situation in a foreign language. It is the role of the simulated patient playing the interpreter to provide most of the learning points. Both may then give competent feedback.

An accurate recording of each simulator's competencies can also inform your future training needs if you are managing your own cohort of simulated patients.

Even if you use an agency and can assume a certain level of training, you may want to consider whether or not the simulated patients would benefit from additional training in order to be effective within your own particular learning environment.

You may have specific feedback requirements or variations on how you wish to manage the session. You may wish to involve the simulated patient more actively or simply to calibrate roles for examination purposes.

Even a small amount of additional training may immeasurably improve your learning outcomes or the validity of your examination.

## DESIGNING A TRAINING PACKAGE

There are so many different aspects to the work that the development of a comprehensive training course for simulated patients is a major undertaking. The breadth and depth of the training you may decide to offer is obviously dependent on the learning objectives of the session/s you are training them to be involved with, the core skill level of the simulated patients you have recruited and, as with everything, the amount of financial resources you have available to you.

I am going to suggest elements that are useful in a simulated patient training course. You may or may not find these relevant to your own objectives, and even if you do find them highly desirable, it is likely that time and resource limitations may require you to cover only the bare essentials. However, with an adequate toolkit of ideas and suggestions, you should be able to make the best of the resources you do have available.

### Introduction

You should establish one basic fact right at the start: simulation is not just acting! It shares some elements with acting but is really quite different, both in its aims and in the skills required. Simulators are not so much actors as reactors. By this I mean that although being a simulated patient involves a degree of performance, it is more about trying to inhabit the skin of the character being played, feeling the things that character may feel and reacting in the way they would react. Simulated patients don't need to be able to mimic exotic accents or project their voice. They don't need to tap-dance or even to know the words of any of Hamlet's soliloquies! Far more important than these 'performance' skills is the ability to see themselves as learning tools and to focus every thought and action on giving the practitioners the opportunity to develop their consultation skills.

You need to give an overview of the work, your personal expectations of a simulated patient and the expectations of the organisation for which they will be working. Many simulated patients work for a variety of organisations, not even necessarily within the healthcare sector. It is essential that they understand the broad principles of the work that they may be embarking on and the aims of the organisation they are working for. This would include the type and experience level of the practitioners and the overall aims of the teaching sessions they are likely to be involved with. If you will be requiring them to take part in different kinds of work (e.g. undergraduate teaching sessions and examinations or one-to-one work and forum sessions), you need to be clear about the demands of each.

You should, if possible, demonstrate a 'typical' session, using more experienced simulated patients, practitioners (or simulated practitioners) and yourself. This demonstration should illustrate the basic principles such as the process, the role portrayal and the giving of constructive feedback. If you are training simulated patients for a specific task, then your demonstration should reflect this. For example, if you are training for examination purposes, you may choose to do three brief demonstrations, to illustrate the chunking of information, the techniques and judgements required to ensure consistency, and the potential pitfalls of the simulated patient who gives all the information out in one go or who overacts their symptoms. If it is not possible to provide a demonstration, you may choose to find a recording of a simulated patient session to demonstrate the basic principles of the work. However, if you choose this option, you should be careful that the recording reflects your own anticipated session/s, or be ready to identify features that do not reflect this. It may be worth considering the possibility of making your own standard recording that can be used repeatedly, if you envisage training more simulated patients in the future.

**Interpreting the brief**
If possible you should send a typical scenario brief (*see* Appendix 2) prior to the training day and ask them to consider how they might develop this before they come. These scenarios can then be worked with, in various ways, during the training session.

This gives you the opportunity to demonstrate how a simulated patient can work with the information given in the brief. Obviously, if you are writing the briefs yourself, you will have responsibility for the quality of these, and you will write them in an unambiguous way. However, if you are expecting them to work with scenario briefs from other sources, you should give the simulated patients some guidance on how to interpret the widely varying standard of content.

In particular, they should always be sure they understand the character's relevant medical history, as they may well be asked for details of this. This should include an understanding of the clinical content and context, not only in terms of specific illnesses and operations they may have had in the past but also in terms of symptoms, treatments, timescales and impact on life. Clearly this may not be relevant in every case, but they should always think about which things may be important, and whether or not they have adequate information.

Also, they should be sure of relevant facts in the character's social situation. Sometimes the social circumstances of the character are largely irrelevant to the scenario; at other times they may be crucial in order to bring out certain teaching points. If a specific type of employment is mentioned in the brief, this may be because some of the duties involved in this particular work may have an impact on the character's symptoms or implications for the future. If this is the case it is important that they have some understanding of this type of employment.

Finally, they should be sure of the aims and objectives of the session and the role of their particular character within that. This may be clear from the brief or the title of the session. If the session is designed to help the practitioners learn how to explain a procedure, for example, the simulated patient should know what sort of questions they should ask and what the level of their character's knowledge is.

### *Always encourage them: if in doubt, ASK!*

The following list is of suggested questions that you could give the trainee simulated patients to make sure they are comfortable with the information they have been given. Obviously, the questions may not all be relevant to the particular scenario they are learning, and some of the information may be deliberately left for them to develop themselves. A quick look through, however, can help them identify any omissions that could be essential to the role and will save them from some potentially stressful improvisation and ad-libbing during the consultation!

➤ Do you have a name?
➤ How old are you?
➤ What is your ethnic and cultural background?
➤ What is your social situation? What is your family life like?
➤ Are you married/single/divorced?
➤ Do you have any children and, if so, how many? Are they girls or boys? How old are they?
➤ Do you work? Where? What is it like?
➤ What is the reason for this interaction? Who initiated it?
➤ What is the background of the current situation?
➤ How would the symptoms be described?
➤ Where is the pain?
➤ When did it begin?
➤ How did it begin? Did anything precipitate it? Was it a sudden or gradual onset?
➤ What is the pain like?
➤ Is the pain just in one place or can you feel it anywhere else?
➤ Are there any other symptoms?

➤ How long does it last each time it comes?
➤ What time of day does it come? Is it constant? How long does it last each time it is there?
➤ Does anything make it worse or better?
➤ How severe are the symptoms?
➤ What are your ideas about what is causing the symptoms?
➤ What are your main worries? Are they around the symptoms and what's causing them, or do you have other concerns that are more pressing?
➤ What are you hoping the outcome of this interaction will be?
➤ What sort of temperament do you have?
➤ What kind of mood are you in as you enter this interaction with the practitioner?
➤ How receptive are you likely to be to the communications of the practitioner? How will you respond to their questions and ideas?
➤ How will you behave during this interaction?
➤ Will your behaviour change? What is likely to make your behaviour change?
➤ Are there any specific parts of the brief that are unclear?
➤ Are there any specific parts of the brief that seem irrelevant to you?

Once they are sure they have all their facts and essential details straight in their minds, they should read through the scenario with a view to getting into role.

When reading the scenario brief, they need to note any important features of the character that may be relevant. Generally speaking, if it is mentioned in the brief, they should remember it. However, if they were to feel that any aspect of the brief was inappropriate for any reason, they should be encouraged to discuss this with the training provider and/or facilitator prior to the session.

The simulator then needs to flesh out the role to create a realistic character that will withstand fairly detailed questioning and a variety of situations. Inevitably each simulated patient will find his or her own favourite techniques for doing this. You may like to give new simulators the following list of suggestions.

➤ They may find it helpful to write copious notes about the character and their social situation.
➤ If there is no timeline given with the scenario, they may find it useful to write one for themselves, to make sure they have an accurate view of what has happened to their character. This is especially helpful if this interaction is the latest in a series of consultations and procedures. For example:
  — 6 months ago began to notice increase in incidence of indigestion
  — 5 months ago went to GP – advised to take antacids
  — 3 months ago returned to GP (symptoms getting worse) – referred to outpatients for investigations
  — 2 weeks ago – called GP as had not received an appointment
  — 1 week ago – attended outpatients for investigations.
➤ They may wish to research any medical conditions on the Internet. This

is useful if they are trying to understand how they might feel about the symptoms they are supposed to be encountering. You should warn them, however, not to include any symptoms that are not mentioned in the brief, unless they have checked with their facilitator first.
➤ Online forums can also help them to understand how a person suffering with certain conditions, or in certain situations, may be feeling.

## Characterisation
### *Getting into role*

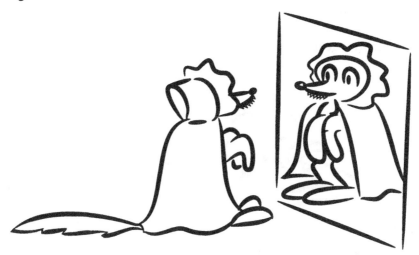

**'All the better to help you to improve your consultation skills my dear!'**

The first thing to do when helping the prospective simulated patients learn how to develop a role is to perform a relevant warm-up. The following is an outline of a useful warm-up for helping prepare people for character building:
➤ Ask everyone to walk around the room. At a given signal they are to stop moving and start a conversation with the person nearest to them.
➤ They should introduce themselves to their partner and tell them two interesting facts about themselves.
➤ One of the things they tell them should be true and the other should be a complete lie.
➤ Their partner can ask questions about their interesting facts in order to gain further information.
➤ After a while everyone should guess which of their partner's interesting facts is true and which is a complete fabrication.
➤ This is a useful introduction to the fact that a simulated patient spends a fair amount of time making up completely false information in order to portray a role convincingly, and they need to uphold this 'lie' under close questioning!

You should encourage them to develop their characters at home. They may choose to spend hours in front of the mirror posing and practising! By doing this they can get a good idea of how they will come across. They can practise responses and reactions. They can assess the extent to which their body language portrays an emotion.

They may simply become that person for a while. They could try to encounter daily life as they imagine that their character would. They can talk, walk and breathe as their character would. If I am working as a simulated patient I often find I chunter away to myself, in role, on the way to work. This helps me to feel focused when I arrive and it brings all the aspects of the character I have developed to the front of my mind. (This, of course, is fine when I am driving but I do get some strange looks if I am on the train!)

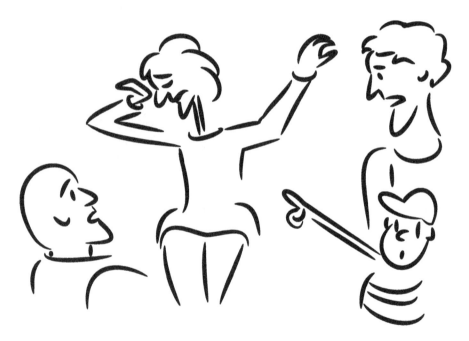

**'Mummy, look at the funny lady . . .!'**

You should think about discussing clothing as an aid to characterisation that the simulated patients may find useful. I am not suggesting that they need a wardrobe extension to house their costume collection, but I think there is little doubt that the clothes a person wears can affect how they feel. If the simulated patient is playing a depressed character, they may want to avoid wearing their smartest clothes; if they are playing an aggressive drug addict, they may not find those padded shoulders and that lipstick too helpful when trying to get into role!

They may also find accessories can be useful. A mobile phone, a half-smoked (unlit!) roll-up, a walking stick . . . encourage them to try different props to see if the props help them to feel more like the person they are trying to portray.

One colleague will simply change his glasses to play a particular character with psychosis. Most people would honestly never notice the difference, but when he wears these other glasses it makes him feel different, so they help him to really get into the skin of the character he is portraying.

However, you should warn the simulated patients to avoid falling into the trap of stereotyping characters! Clothing and accessories are simply an aid to help *them* to get into role, to be able to feel as though they are giving a realistic portrayal of the character they are portraying. I am not in any way suggesting that there are no smartly dressed heroin users or magistrates who wear combat trousers!

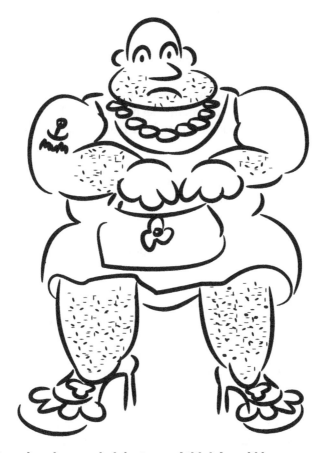

**'I've missed my period doctor . . . I think I could be pregnant!'**

### Building up the character
It may then be useful to do some character development exercises in the group. The following is an example of a useful activity to help trainees get into role.

➤ Give everyone a brief character outline, possibly with some indication of mood. For example:

'You are a football supporter, going to watch your local team play, for the first time ever, at Wembley.'

'You are a stressed businessman/woman going to an important meeting.'

'You are an impoverished student going to visit a feared elderly relative to try to secure a loan.'

➤ Tell them they are passengers on a coach travelling to London that has broken down. They have been ushered into a room in a motorway service area to wait while the situation is assessed.
➤ Ask them to interact with the other passengers in the roles you have assigned to them.
➤ After a while you could give additional information such as further delays, cancellation, arrival of replacement coach and so forth.
➤ Freeze the action at various points to hear from different people how they are feeling (in role).

Another very useful exercise is 'hot-seating'. One use of hot-seating is described later, in Chapter 9, where we see how it can be used to quickly gather information about a patient, within a teaching situation. However, hot-seating, as used for developing a character, is slightly different, so I will describe it briefly. Although the simulated patient will not have the opportunity to hot-seat every role that they play, they can adapt the technique in a DIY way to help in the development of characters.

For this exercise, you can use the same scenario you sent out before the train-ing session, or you can simply give a brief outline of a character. The person who is to be hot-seated tries to get into role using the information they have been given. They then sit in front of the rest of the group (in the hot seat) and the group asks them questions about absolutely anything.

'Do you live alone? ... Do you have children? ... What are their names? ... Where do you work? ... Do you enjoy work? ... What sort of house do you live in? ... Are you a tidy person? ... What newspaper do you read? ... Where did you go on holiday last year? ... Do you have any pets? ... How did you vote in the last election? ... Are you faithful to your partner? ... What is your date of birth? ... What time did you go to bed last night? ... What is your favourite drink? ... If you were a piece of furniture, what would you be? ... When was the last time you cried? ... What is the name of your local pub?'

The questions should be fired as quickly as possible. The act of trying to answer the questions as the character they are portraying would answer them is a very effective way of developing a realistic character. It also gives the simulated patient good practice in thinking up answers to unprepared questions. It doesn't really matter how the simulated patients develop their characters – everyone will find ways they find more effective than others. The important thing is that they are prepared and able to feel, to the best of their ability, how the character they are portraying is feeling. In this way they will be able to react more appropriately and they will be able to give more useful and sensitive feedback to the practitioner.

### *Varying the role*

While the simulated patients are preparing their roles, it is also worth encouraging them to think about different ways in which they could vary the scenario. They may only need to play the role once, but there may be times when it would be useful to be able to ask them to play it several times and with variations depending on the needs of the group of learners. It is useful to give the simulators a repertoire of methods by which they can alter the role they are playing, perhaps to increase the complexity of the scenario or to make it more straightforward, perhaps to alter the focus or simply to provide variety within a session.

Ask them to think of the character they are playing and imagine what would happen if:
➤ their medical condition had worsened or improved . . . how would that change their behaviour?
➤ their social situation had changed . . . how would their character face redundancy, promotion, separation, bereavement?
➤ they were in a different mood? What moods might they be capable of? The mood of a patient varies and therefore so must the mood of the simulated patient.
➤ they were shy? Ask them to try to imagine a shy version of the same character, or a very garrulous one. What if they were more or less assertive?

These are just suggestions to generate ideas. Invite them to be as creative as they like with this to help prepare them for possible situations that may require a variation of their role. Reassure them that when they gain more experience, adjusting their portrayal of the role will become much easier. The situation itself may allow for variations. For example, if they are referred for some investigations at the hospital, this may carry different outcomes and therefore an opportunity for different reactions. Insist that the simulated patients always check out their ideas for a variation with you or their facilitator before using them in a session.

You should reassure them that if, however, they felt that they were unable to portray the character in the way that you, or the facilitator, were asking for, they should be given the opportunity to discuss alternatives. There are usually a variety of ways to achieve the same learning outcomes, and it is preferable to have a simulated patient who is confident in their role rather than one who may feel awkward and therefore play it in a way that compromises the learning objectives.

### Altering the role

You should warn the simulated patients that occasionally they may be asked to completely alter the scenario if there is a particular learning point that you or another facilitator or, indeed, the practitioners themselves wish to explore or emphasise. Explain that this may arise from the previous session, or from something that has happened during the current session, and that there is really no planning for this situation. A simulated patient simply needs to be flexible and creative and generally wonderful!

However, again, you should advise them to take the time to discuss the situation with the facilitator to ensure they feel confident that they are able to meet the needs of the group. The discussion may have to be brief, a few moments only, before they begin the scenario.

Ask them to make sure they feel confident with the situation. Tell them they should not be afraid to say no. If they feel uncomfortable for any reason with something they have been asked to do, they should try to talk about it. The situation may be easily resolved by a few minor changes. The clearer everyone is about the aims and objectives of the session and their own capabilities, the more successful the outcome is likely to be. However, although it is better if a compromise of some kind can be reached through this discussion with the facilitator, if the facilitator insists they portray a certain role in a certain way, they should endeavour to do so.

Emphasise that if they feel unsure of the facilitator's expectations in any way, they should ask! The development of an effective scenario needs to be by negotiation. The facilitator may well have a clear idea of how they would like a certain role played and it is the simulated patient's responsibility to try to do this to the best of their ability.

### De-roling

Some of the roles simulated patients may be asked to play will be emotionally challenging. You should warn them that occasionally they may be asked to play a role that they feel is too 'close to home'. Once more, I would stress to them the importance of feeling able to refuse. A simulated patient who has been, for example, receiving bad news when in role but remains inconsolable when they are supposed to be giving feedback out of role is less than ideal. I know . . . I have been that simulated patient! I am now very careful to avoid certain scenarios that I know I will find too distressing; however, many simulated patients may not feel they are able to do this. If this is the case, emphasise to them that they should turn down the work at the time they are offered it. It is unfair of them to decide they cannot do a role when they have arrived at a session. Obviously, if it is a practitioner-directed session (*see* Chapter 9) this will not be an option, as there is no way of knowing what challenging issues the practitioners will bring.

Once more, encourage them to negotiate a situation that they feel they can cope with. For example, if it is a session dealing with breaking bad news, often it only takes the alteration of a few social details to protect the simulated patient's feelings while maintaining the integrity of the role and the effectiveness of the learning.

You should stress the importance of de-roling after a session. Often it happens naturally through the discussion and feedback time. Often the role has not been intense enough to cause any problems. Often the feeling of elation that accompanies the realisation that they do not have all the problems of the character they have been playing is enough to lift them back into the real world! Some simulated patients will put on or take off a scarf or jacket, a small symbol, to differentiate between the real them and the simulated one.

Emphasise that the important thing is for them to take a moment to make sure that they have left the character in the consultation and if they have not, to make sure they do something to de-role.

> Once I was playing a heroin user at a Royal College of General Practitioners conference about drug misuse. It was a 'cameo' situation where I was not required to give any feedback out of role. Immediately afterwards we had a coffee break, during which I was approached by one of the speakers, a genuine drug user from the Methadone Alliance. He nudged me and said conspiratorially, 'They try hard this lot but they just don't understand the likes of me and you, do they?' This was one rare occasion when I felt it more appropriate to remain in role for a little while longer!

## GIVING FEEDBACK

*You cannot teach a crab*
*to walk straight!*

Aristophanes (446–386 BC)

One of the most important tasks the simulated patient must perform is also one of the most challenging ... the giving of feedback. While the practitioner will have his or her own impression of how the session went and the observers of the consultation will have their own impressions, it is the simulated patient who perhaps has the best idea of what it really felt like for the patient; this allows a unique opportunity for some insightful feedback.

The giving of feedback, however, is also the part that can leave a practitioner confident and ready to learn or demoralised and ready to give up. Therefore, it is essential that the training the simulated patients receive covers feedback in quite considerable depth, unless they are only required for examinations, where feedback is not required.

Here we will look at how to train the simulated patients to ensure that the receiving of feedback is a positive learning experience for the practitioners. This should also give you a deeper understanding of the different methods of giving feedback and how you can fully utilise them to maximise the positive impact on the practitioners. You should make sure the simulated patients know the purpose of feedback. This is crucial in order for them to give it usefully and constructively.

## Principles

### *Feedback should be honest*

That feedback should be honest does not mean to say that it should not be positive and constructive; however, you should encourage simulated patients to avoid insincerity in their comments. Warn them that this will sometimes lead to moments of panic! A consultation has finished and they cannot think of a single positive thing to say. Tell them to relax at this point . . . to think back to the aims and objectives of the session, to think of the introduction, the way the practitioner was sitting . . . there has to be some positive aspect they can find to comment on.

Tell them that, ideally, they should be hearing comments from the practitioners before they have to make their own, and so this should help prompt them as well as giving them an indication of the state of mind of the practitioner. However, you should warn the simulated patients that although this is the most effective order in which to organise feedback, not all facilitators may know or remember this. Therefore, the simulated patients should be prepared to speak first on occasions. Advise them to be cautious in this situation, perhaps only speaking in positive terms initially until they have managed to gauge the practitioner's own reaction to their consultation.

Remind the simulated patients that their primary function is as a teaching resource. If they are faced with a practitioner who has a very negative view of his or her own performance during the consultation, it would be insensitive to endorse this with their own negative feedback. In this case, it is more helpful for the simulated patient to give as much feedback on the positive things about the session as they can. If there are a lot of things that could have been done differently, recommend that, instead of directing a lot of constructive feedback at the practitioner, they talk about what a difficult situation it was, what a difficult character they played and how well the practitioner did to deal with it at all. Then it may be possible for the simulated patient to give one or two gentle pointers to things that the practitioner may want to consider trying in the future.

The more confident practitioner may be better able to hear constructive feedback from the simulated patient. However, it may be worth giving the simulated patients a word of warning about the arrogant practitioner! Although it is sometimes tempting to be super-critical of practitioners who appear arrogant and cocky, this attitude often masks insecurity; therefore, total annihilation of their protective shell (however unpleasant it may appear to the simulated patient) could be dangerous! In this case, simulated patients should endeavour, as always, to give balanced feedback as they would to anyone else.

Emphasise that their feedback should be honest but not brutal! While maintaining integrity in all they say, they should also remember the point of feedback. It is intended to help a practitioner to identify the skills and attributes they have that are effective, and to explore alternatives to less helpful strategies. Feedback that is not given in the spirit of helping can become destructive and is to be avoided at all costs.

Remind them that they are giving feedback on behaviours, not on personality.

### Feedback should be non-judgemental

It is important that the simulated patients should understand the importance of trying to make their feedback non-judgemental.

You could explain to them that there are no real rights or wrongs in the world of consultation skills training; rather, there is cause and effect. As we have mentioned before, both patients and healthcare practitioners are individuals and because of this, every interaction is unique. As such, every opinion about what is effective communication and what appears less so is entirely subjective. This invalidates any judgemental feedback as it is necessarily merely the perception of one individual.

This said, I think positive 'judgemental' feedback may be acceptable if it is merely being used to cushion the effects of some constructive comments. The important thing is that you make the simulated patients absolutely conscious of the type of feedback they are offering.

### Feedback should be relevant

Feedback needs to be relevant to the aims and objectives of the teaching session and to the level of training at which the practitioners are working, so ask the simulated patients to make sure they know what these are!

Some simulated patients will contribute anecdotes and personal theories or experiences during feedback sessions. These are very occasionally useful in helping to illustrate a point, but more often than not they simply distract the group from its purpose. Ask them to try to limit their feedback to what has actually happened during the session.

### Feedback should be specific and descriptive

General feedback should be avoided if possible. Comments such as

'I thought you were really good'

may be pleasant for the practitioner to hear but are perhaps less helpful than a more specific indication of what it was that the practitioner did that led to that outcome. Encourage them to say, for example,

'When I started to get upset and you put your hand on my arm, it made me feel really comforted and reassured.'

'When you told me I had a hieroglyphic globalotomy I felt really scared . . .'

'The part where you stopped asking me about my symptoms and started asking me about my experiences in London made me feel as though I really wanted to start opening up to you and tell you about what was really bothering me.'

Descriptive feedback gives the practitioner specific examples of those consultation techniques that may be more or less effective. This is sometimes easier to do than others. Often simulated patients will only be expected to answer specific questions from the practitioner, facilitator or group. Examples of this could be:

'How did you feel about me writing notes during the consultation?'

'When I raised the subject of your mother you went quiet and looked upset. Could I have asked the question in another way?'

In this case, it is easy to give specific feedback.

At other times the simulator may be asked for feedback more generally, which makes it more difficult to respond with specific information. It is for situations like this that you should point out the advantages to the trainee simulated patient of understanding some of the different theories and models of feedback. For example, when asked:

'How do you think it went, then?'

it is useful for the simulator to have some ideas about how to give both positive and constructive comments to help the practitioner to further develop their skills.

Some groups will form projections on how they imagine the patient is feeling. In this case, the simulator will need only to confirm, or otherwise, their projections, possibly with some reasoning behind their reaction. For example:

'I think you resented the nurse asking about your work.'

To which they may reply:

'Yes, I did resent it. I think I had already given the reasons quite clearly, why I felt I couldn't go to work. It made me feel as though I wasn't really being listened to.'

It is important also to bear in mind what I call the 'cause and effect' aspect of consultation skills teaching. If a practitioner says something that makes the simulator's character feel angry, for example, this does not necessarily mean there is anything intrinsically wrong with what was said. It is important, therefore, for the simulated patient to stress the character's responses rather than the behaviour of the practitioner. For example, instead of saying,

> 'When you talked about the operation you were a bit dismissive of my fears'

they could say:

> 'I felt quite upset and anxious when you described the operation so quickly . . . I would have liked to have been given a bit more time to talk about the things I feel scared about.'

### Address feedback directly to the practitioner

Explain to the simulated patients that although this may sound straightforward, when asked direct questions by the facilitator or group members it may sometimes seem awkward or inappropriate to address replies to the practitioner who has carried out the consultation. However, it is more direct and therefore more powerful for the simulated patient to give their feedback directly to the consulting practitioner. They will, however, as always, need to remain flexible and respond to each situation accordingly. There are occasions when the power of giving direct feedback to the practitioner (while giving constructive feedback) may be too great. This will be looked at in more detail in Chapter 11.

You should also ensure that the simulated patients are aware of the potential impact of feedback they give.

### Feedback warm-up

The effects of constructive and destructive feedback can be illustrated very effectively using the following exercise.
➤ Get five volunteers from the group to come and stand at the front.
➤ Divide the rest of the participants into five groups and allocate each group a volunteer to observe.
➤ Ask the volunteers to perform a task – this can be anything but should be brief. For example, you could ask them to 'barrel roll', which involves:
  – first rotating their right arm away from their body
  – then rotating their left arm towards their body
  – then rotating both arms simultaneously – right arm away, left arm towards – for a few moments and then ask them to stop. (It is more effective if you practise this task beforehand so that you can do it with ease!)

➤ Walk along the line of people, from one to five, with the following comments:
  — You are rubbish.
  — That wasn't very good.
  — You need to work on your barrel rolling.
  — How do you think that went? (Get an answer but say nothing further)
  — How do you think that went? (Respond to their answer with a discussion, encouraging them to think of ways of improving their barrel-rolling skills.)
➤ Discuss with the group the effects of each form of feedback on the volunteers.

This exercise can also be done with an easier activity and different degrees of positive feedback, in order to demonstrate how unhelpful non-descriptive, non-specific feedback is, even when it is supposed to be positive and encouraging.

### Gathering points to give feedback on

You should discuss the challenge of gathering points to give feedback on. This is a difficult process for the simulated patient. While everyone else in the group is taking careful notes and focusing completely and critically on the interaction, the simulated patient is trying to give a realistic portrayal of a character as well as trying to respond appropriately and constructively to questions. On top of this, through careful observation of the practitioner's behaviour, both verbal and non-verbal, and a close monitoring of the effects this behaviour has on their character's feelings, they must gather appropriate comments to make at the end, in order to assist the practitioner in improving and developing their consultation skills techniques. This is certainly not an easy task!

It illustrates one of the main differences between acting and simulation. Remind them that it is important not to get so carried away in the performance that they fail to observe the interaction between the two people concerned – their character and the practitioner. It is within this interaction that the learning takes place, so it is vital that they monitor it closely.

There are no hard and fast rules about how to teach them to do this. Some people find it easier to form a structure in their head; for example, one colleague chooses a point from the beginning, from the middle and from the end of the consultation. Another makes a mental note as soon as possible in the consultation of one good point and one behaviour that could be tried differently. It is really up to the simulated patient to try different methods of remembering points.

You, of course, as facilitator in the teaching session, will order the feedback in such a way that the simulated patient will hear the viewpoints of the practitioner and the other members of the group first. This is essential for the simulator. It can help if their mind goes blank and they cannot think of a thing to say (as happens to everybody at some time). It can also help to let them know at what level to pitch their feedback. This is explored in more depth in Chapter 11. It also affords the opportunity to listen to the points that are raised during feedback, as they can then add their viewpoint to those already mentioned and often they can evidence the observations made by the practitioner, facilitator and group. This adds coherence, meaning and structure to the session.

### What sort of things will they need to give feedback on?

Each practitioner is unique, as is each simulated patient. Therefore, each interaction is also unique and so the range of behaviours and feelings a simulated patient could potentially give feedback on is infinite.

You may like to give the simulated patients the following list of possible topics for feedback, but encourage them not to feel limited by this – it is only meant as a guide. Equally, they should not feel the need to include all of these topics. Sometimes it may only be appropriate to give one piece of feedback, but at other times a more overall or detailed approach will be needed.

➤ How were you greeted? Formally? Informally? Did they smile? How did their introduction make you feel?

➤ Did you feel the practitioner had arranged the furniture in a way that made you feel comfortable? Were the seats so close that you felt your personal space was invaded or were you so far apart that it made it difficult to hear?

➤ Did the practitioner introduce himself or herself politely? Did you know their name and what their role was? Did you know the reason for the interaction you were about to have?

➤ Did they check your name and ask how you would like to be addressed? If not, how did it make you feel to be addressed by your first name, for example?

➤ If you have come to the consultation with a relative or interpreter, did the practitioner manage to welcome you both politely?

➤ During the interaction, did the practitioner seem interested in you? How did you know whether or not they were?

➤ How were they sitting? Leaning forwards or backwards? How did it make you feel?

➤ Did they appear to be calm and confident or were they nervously fidgeting with their hands, pen and so forth?

➤ Did they seem to be listening to what you were saying? How did you know whether or not they were? Maybe they were nodding, or using encouraging sounds such as 'aha . . . mmm . . .'? Maybe they summarised what you were saying?

➤ What was their tone of voice like?

➤ Did you understand everything the practitioner said to you? If not, why not? Were they using medical jargon, or simply not adjusting their vocabulary to match that of the character you were playing?

➤ Did you feel that the practitioner cared about you? If so, how did you know? Was it simply the expression on their face, or was it the words they used?

➤ Did the practitioner touch you at any point? If so, was it appropriate or did it make you feel uncomfortable?

➤ Did you feel that you had enough time and encouragement to tell the practitioner all that you wanted to tell them? Did the pace of the consultation feel fast, slow or just right?

➤ Did you get to discuss any options for treatment suggested by the practitioner, or did they just tell you what they felt would be best?

➤ Did the practitioner seem professional?

➤ Did it feel as though there was an order to the consultation, or did you jump from topic to topic? Did you know why questions were being asked or did it sometimes seem quite random?

➤ Did they know that you know what they know?! Did you feel that the practitioner made sure that you understood what had been discussed and what was going to happen?

➤ Were there any particularly significant moments? Sometimes when simulated patients are in role, something the practitioner says or does can have a real impact on them. It can sometimes be difficult to put it into words, but can be very powerful feedback.

➤ Do you trust the practitioner you have seen? Would you choose to come back to see them?

> Recently I was playing a brash and very talkative character who had been living on the streets for many years. The student carrying out the consultation suddenly asked me if I felt lonely. Since the discussion until that point had been focused very much on whether or not she was going to prescribe me some benzodiazepines, the question completely took me by surprise. It also made a fundamental shift in the relationship between the character and the student. This was difficult to describe because it made the character feel unusually cared for, but it also made her feel a little exposed and therefore vulnerable. It was a powerful moment, and was a turning point in the consultation and brought some interesting discussion during out-of-role feedback.

**The great in-role/out-of-role debate**

More information is given in Chapter 11 on how to use in-role and out-of-role feedback and when it is appropriate to have the simulated patient be role neutral within a teaching session. Here we will focus on how to train the simulators to do them all.

First of all, you need to teach the simulated patients the difference between giving feedback in role, out of role and in role neutral.

In-role feedback is the feedback given when they are still playing the part of the character portrayed in the consultation. They should respond as their character would respond to any questions asked.

Out-of-role feedback is the feedback they give after the facilitator has invited them to come out of role. They should then be responding to questions as themselves.

Role neutral is simply a term I use to describe dispassionate in-role feedback. Often the simulated patients may be asked to give feedback in role but without any of the strong emotions that may have been evident during the consultation. It is a subtle and sophisticated technique that involves them imagining their character in a less emotionally charged situation. It is similar to the level of characterisation required for hot-seating, as described earlier in this chapter.

You should explain that there is an element of role neutral in all in-role feedback, since the focus of the conversation shifts considerably at the end of a consultation. Instead of a one-to-one interaction, in which the well-being of the patient is the primary subject, the simulated patient's character is now involved in a group discussion about the practitioner and their skills.

You should stress to the trainee simulated patients the importance of remaining clear in their own minds whether they are in role or out of role when they are giving their feedback.

Very occasionally, they may be invited to come out of role to give feedback and take part in the group discussion and then be asked to go back into role to replay a certain part or move the consultation on to a different stage. This can be a little difficult sometimes. The simulated patient should take a few moments to reflect on the character they have been playing, the situation they have been in and the feedback and discussion they have heard and participated in. They may be required to initiate proceedings or the practitioner may reopen the interview. They should follow the lead of the facilitator, who will hopefully be clear about the expectations.

Simulated patients may initially find it a bit confusing and difficult to differentiate between giving feedback in or out of role. This is easier at some times than others. If they have been playing a character that is far removed from their own, it is often easier to distinguish in-role from out-of-role feedback. It is more difficult if the character they have been playing is similar in temperament, situation or outlook to their own.

One technique you may find useful to share with them is for them to speak in the first person (obviously!) as the patient but to refer to the patient in the third person when they are out of role. So when speaking as the patient, they may say:

'I felt really comforted when you just touched my arm.'

When speaking out of role they could say:

'She felt very comforted when you just touched her arm.'

'Sonja felt very comforted when you just touched her arm.'

This allows for a certain detachment and gives clarity to everyone as to whether the simulator is in or out of role.

### Qualitative differences among in-role, out-of-role and role-neutral feedback

It may also be useful to ask the trainee simulated patients to briefly consider the qualitative differences among these methods of giving feedback.

If they were to reflect on, for example, a practitioner's use of eye contact, feedback given in role may be:

> 'The way you kept on looking at me made me feel like you were really interested in what I was trying to say.'

Feedback given out of role may be:

> 'You maintained good eye contact throughout.'

Similarly, if they were to comment on the practitioner's use of silence, they may say in role:

> 'Occasionally I felt like I was just about to say something and then you asked me another question so I forgot what I was going to say ... like when you asked me about my mother, and before I had had much time to think, asked me how many times I went to see her each day.'

Out of role they may say:

> 'You may want to think about your use of silence ... Amy would probably have told you more if you had left slightly more space for her to speak.'

They may then go on to talk about other specific examples from within the consultation.

An example of giving role-neutral feedback if, for instance, the simulated patient has been crying in role, may be:

> 'It made me feel as though you really did care about me when you touched my arm as I started to cry.'

This should be said without tears and extreme emotion, although still obviously sad.

Similarly, if they have been extremely frustrated or angry in role, they may say something like:

> 'Yeah, well, I suppose you was only trying to help when you offered me someone else to talk to . . . but I really wasn't happy about it . . . it felt like you was just palming me off.'

This could be said in a grumpy tone but not with the same levels of frustration or rudeness that may have been used during the consultation.

## Constructive feedback

Emphasise to the simulated patients that the way in which they give constructive feedback is crucial. This is the greatest responsibility the simulated patients have. A practitioner's confidence can be completely undermined or even destroyed by the receiving of insensitive feedback.

Obviously, it is easier to give feedback on the aspects a practitioner has performed effectively. Giving guidance about behaviours they may wish to alter or develop differently is altogether more challenging. Just as the practitioners are learning techniques to become more effective in their consultation, so the simulated patient must learn techniques to give constructive or less positive feedback effectively.

The following are some suggestions you can give to the trainee simulated patients – again, not an exhaustive list – of some strategies for making their constructive feedback a positive experience for the practitioner.

### Make feedback descriptive

Making feedback descriptive has been mentioned before, but simply describing a behaviour can be more effective than criticising the behaviour.

Compare

> 'You shouldn't have stared at the computer screen when you were talking to me.'

with

> 'You started to type on the computer while I was telling you about my husband's moods.'

The simulated patients can also describe the feelings that they experienced as a result of certain behaviours. For example:

> 'I did feel rather upset when you started to type on the computer while I was telling you about my husband's moods. It felt as though you weren't really listening to me.'

### Word all comments carefully

It is often possible to take a criticism and word it in such a way that it sounds like a helpful suggestion.

Compare

'You were right in my face, really invading my personal body space.'

with

'It may have been helpful to have arranged the seating in such a way that there was a wider space between us.'

### Link with a positive

If the simulated patient can link their comment with a piece of positive feedback, it seems less like a major criticism and more like a minor adjustment that could be made to improve the consultation.

Compare

'You asked me what I thought then didn't let me speak.'

with

'It was great the way you asked me for my ideas on the possible causes of my symptoms . . . it would have been even better though, if you could have left a little more space afterwards for me to think about it and give my answers.'

### Give effects of behaviours

The simulated patient should try to help the practitioner to understand exactly what the patient's difficulty was with any given behaviour, and what the consequences could be, if any, for the practitioner. For example:

'When you asked me all those questions in a row, I wasn't sure which one I should answer . . . I think I ended up only answering the last one you asked . . . which I suppose means you never did find out about my sleeping problems.'

### Suggest alternatives

If the simulated patient can suggest other ways the practitioner could try to tackle a problem, this is often more helpful than simply criticising the behaviour. Point out to the simulated patients that it is mainly the job of the facilitator to encourage the practitioner and the group to come up with suggestions, as that is how they will best learn, but that sometimes it may be helpful for the simulator to offer alternatives. For example:

> 'When you were explaining to me what you thought the best thing to do next would be, you seemed to talk about an awful lot of things . . . I think I got a bit lost, really. I suppose it might have helped if you could have just tried to tell me one thing at a time.'

### Avoid imperatives

There are no real rights or wrongs about consultation techniques, just more or less effective strategies. Therefore, it is seldom appropriate to say:

> 'You must . . .'

> 'You should . . .'

> 'You need to . . .'

It is better to soften any suggestions you have by using the following:

> 'You may want to try . . .'

> 'You could . . .'

> 'It may be worth . . .'

### Use an in-role/out-of-role combination

Experienced simulated patients can also use the opportunities offered by their character to give less palatable feedback, tempered by the feedback they later give out of role. For example, if asked by a practitioner how the patient feels about them at the end of a consultation, the simulator may say in role:

> 'You're a bleeding arrogant middle-class twit who should be struck off the register!'

They may then make it less harsh and more constructive during out-of-role feedback by saying:

> 'Obviously she was disgruntled by your refusal to give her what she wanted. She is quite clearly not the easiest person in the world to get on with. I think anyone would have struggled with that . . . I was wondering

though . . . perhaps if you had taken a little more time at the beginning of the consultation to try to understand some of her social difficulties she may have felt less alienated by the end.'

## Ongoing feedback

You should encourage the simulated patients to be aware of the overt reactions they show during the consultation, and to develop this awareness to enable them to use it as a technique to give the practitioner ongoing feedback throughout the interaction. Ongoing feedback is a term I use to describe spontaneous responses that are given during the course of a consultation. It is simply the reaction of the simulated patient to what is going on. Ongoing feedback may be verbal, but more commonly it is non-verbal responses that help the practitioner recognise how their communications are being received.

For example, if a practitioner casually and dismissively mentions a potential diagnosis that the patient was not expecting, the simulator should respond, either verbally or non-verbally, to indicate their surprise or distress. This gives the practitioner the chance to address their concerns and restore the rapport that they have been trying to build.

This is an often unacknowledged method of giving feedback, but it is one that is very important for the simulated patient to remain aware of at all times. It is also one of the major differences between being an actor and being a teaching resource. As the simulated patient gets into role and inhabits a particular character, it is easy to (and important not to) forget the main purpose of the exercise.

If, for example, they are playing an upset/frustrated/angry patient and the practitioner uses effective consultation techniques, it is important for them to consider whether or not to reflect that back during the consultation. Is it appropriate to become less upset/frustrated/angry, or would this be totally unrealistic for the sort of character they are playing? In reality, perhaps the particular character would not be able to regain control over their behaviour; however, this is a teaching situation, and it may be more helpful to give a positive response to positive techniques.

If the simulated patient decides not to respond during the consultation (which may occasionally be appropriate), then it is important that they explain this during feedback and acknowledge the practitioner's skills nonetheless.

They may say, for example:

> 'With all the experiences that Martin has had recently with the healthcare system, I think it would have taken a lot more than you could possibly have done in this one difficult consultation to calm him down. Having said that, however, you made a fantastic effort! I think when Martin goes home and thinks about today, he is very likely to make another appointment to see you, because you were showing such empathy and sensitivity to his situation that, despite himself, he was beginning to warm to you.'

It is absolutely crucial, as I have stressed before, that you make sure the simulated patients master the art of giving potentially difficult feedback in a way that the practitioner can understand as a means to help them develop their skills, rather than it being seen as a destructive experience.

### Written feedback

Simulated patients are occasionally required to give written feedback to or about practitioners.

This may, for example, be following a consultation within an assessment setting. Explain to them that usually they are given a structure to follow within this; for example, a series of specific questions to answer.

They may also be asked to give written feedback within a teaching situation, whereby they may be asked either to answer specific questions or to give more generalised feedback. For example, they may be asked to provide three examples of behaviours demonstrated by the student that helped the patient to feel comfortable within the consultation and three examples of behaviours that were less helpful.

They should always find out and be clear about whether they are supposed to be writing their feedback in or out of role and exactly what is expected from this written feedback. It is a subtle difference, but if asked to write feedback in role, they should view it very much as they would if they were giving verbal feedback in role neutral. If they are in role, they are still describing how they were feeling and what they think the practitioner or candidate was doing to make them feel that way. The focus should be very much on the behaviour of the practitioner or candidate, rather than the outcome of the consultation, and on the effect that the behaviour had on the patient. It is more straightforward when they are writing out of role and it is easier for the simulated patient to make a more objective assessment, using consultation skills terminology.

Remind the simulated patient to be descriptive and specific in their written feedback, just as they should be when giving verbal feedback. If they make a statement about how a particular part of the consultation made the patient feel, they should make sure they back it up with specific evidence from the consultation. This gives context and clarity to their feedback.

### Practice

Finally, in a training session for simulated patients, you should allow plenty of time for all trainees to practise. Based on the wise words of Confucius cited at the beginning of this book, we should follow the same principle of actually doing, rather than simply hearing or seeing. Experience is far more beneficial to the learning process than witnessing.

They should have the opportunity to practise creating a role, giving information and giving feedback. How you organise these practice sessions depends very much on your resources. Ideally you would divide them into very small groups and allocate a practitioner to each pair or group of three. They could then practise the skills needed to be an effective simulated patient while having a realistic interaction with a practitioner. It would also allow for the practitioner to give them some feedback on the experience from their perspective. However, it is rare for an organisation to be able to fund this, although you may be able to persuade students to participate for a very small remuneration, as they may appreciate the extra experience.

If you have any experienced simulated patients, they could take the part of the practitioners in the groups, although you will probably face a similar resource problem.

In the absence of a practitioner, student or experienced simulated patient for each group, you could divide them into groups of three or four, with one person taking the part of the practitioner, another practising the skills of the simulated patient, and the other one or two as observers. They should swap roles regularly until everyone has had a turn at each role. The main problem with using inexperienced simulated patients as practitioners is that they often are not sure of the sorts of questions they should be asking.

You could ease this process by writing a list of suggested areas of questioning, or even actual basic questions, according to which groups of practitioners you envisage the simulated patients working with. These could be on a flip chart placed just within sight of the trainee asking the questions, so they could refer to it if they cannot think of what to ask.

### Situations that may require specialist training

If your requirements are more specific, it is useful to offer further training on top of this.

### Portraying characters with mental health problems

If you need the simulated patients to present more complex mental health scenarios, it is worth offering some extra guidance on this. Some mental health roles are particularly challenging for many simulated patients. Most people have experienced a range of physical symptoms such as pain, itchiness, fatigue or stiffness. Simulated patients can usually, therefore, draw on their own experiences to guess how the patients they are portraying may be feeling, even if they have not suffered from the exact condition they are endeavouring to present.

However, with mental health scenarios, fewer people have experienced, for example, the auditory or visual hallucinations characteristic of a psychotic illness, or the extreme confusion that can be seen in people with dementia. Therefore, if you ask a simulated patient to portray a person who is suffering with mental health difficulties, you should try to help them gain some insight into what it is like to have such symptoms. This could be in the form of general training about portraying people with various symptoms of mental distress. It could also be in the form of working up specific roles.

If it is not possible, for whatever reason, to offer a dedicated mental health training session for the simulated patients, it is important that you find a way to give them an idea of how the character they will be portraying experiences life, in order that they can give a reasonable presentation of some of the problems faced. There are a number of ways in which you can do this.

➤ Offering the opportunity to talk with people who have experienced the particular mental health difficulty you are asking the simulated patient to portray is probably the most effective way for them to gain some insight. This is not often an option, for many practical and ethical reasons. It is probably less problematic to find a healthcare professional who has some experience of working with people suffering from mental health difficulties, to get their view of the problems the simulated patient's character may be facing.

➤ There are also many portrayals in the arts, in many forms (e.g. literature, film, art, poetry) of people who are suffering from mental health problems. By reading poems or stories or watching films, for example, simulators can gain very sensitive insights into what it may be like to live with some of the problems faced by people with different kinds of mental health difficulties. You could suggest possible sources of insights within the arts, as there are as many unrealistic, unhelpful or too extreme portrayals of people suffering with mental health difficulties in the media. Some suggestions for useful resources are found in Appendix 3.

➤ You could direct them to useful books or websites that clarify issues around the lives of people with mental health problems.

➤ You could simply talk with the simulated patient, giving an outline of the kinds of feelings the patient might have, the kinds of phenomena they may be experiencing and the kinds of behaviour they may be exhibiting.

### Bilingual simulated patients

In our increasingly multicultural society, the challenges health professionals face in communicating with people whose first language is not English grow ever more complex. Simulated patients can be very useful to present and explore some of the issues such consultations may present to both the health professional and the patient, and also to the interpreter if one is used.

If you are planning to work with bilingual simulated patients, they will need additional training as the process in these sessions is often more complex. It is also less likely that many of the bilingual simulated patients you are able to recruit will have a specific background in drama, and so may lack confidence in portraying characters too far from their own. This tendency should be reflected in the training you offer.

The following warm-up is not only useful for training bilingual simulated patients but also very useful as a warm-up for the practitioners in the session as it clearly illustrates some of the difficulties inherent in consultations where language presents a barrier to communication.

On separate cards, write out a series of different reasons why a patient may decide to visit a general practitioner. To be most effective in this exercise, it is useful to include in each one element that is relatively easy to portray and another that is less obviously so.

Examples may include:

> 'You have been off work with a bad backache and are concerned about your job security.'

> 'You have been getting headaches for about 3 months now, and you are worried as a work colleague recently died of a brain tumour.'

> 'You have come about your husband, who seems to be getting increasingly forgetful.'

Give a 'symptom' to each trainee and ask them, in pairs, to convey what is written on their card to their partner without using any words. You can allow the listener to ask questions to clarify what the other is trying to say, which is challenging enough in itself. If you feel like being really cruel and making the challenge even more realistic, you can forbid any conversation at all until the end of each turn, when the listener has to guess what their partner's problem is.

Not only is this great fun and a very effective ice-breaker but also it gives the trainees (or practitioners in a teaching session) an insight into the frustrations of trying to make oneself understood and of trying to understand each other without a common language.

If you are recruiting and training bilingual simulators, it is often useful to do so in 'language pairs'. This enables a stronger working relationship to be developed between the simulated patients who will be working together, although you must remember that they may not always be available at the same time.

An effective way of training bilingual simulated patients that not only accommodates the personal attributes of the trainees but also usefully incorporates significant cultural elements that may be appropriate to explore in a session is to develop the roles that you will be using with the trainees themselves. By clearly outlining the anticipated learning points, it is often then possible and most useful to ask the trainees to work up a scenario between language pairs/language groups. This ensures that the scenarios that are developed can be confidently presented by the simulated patients you are working with; it also highlights certain cultural issues that may present themselves. As the learning points in these sessions tend to focus on communication issues, the clinical details may often be less relevant, although clearly such information must be checked by a clinician and accurately presented to enable diagnosis if needed.

As well as developing the details of the scenario, it is also useful in training to explore issues around cultural behaviour and ways of maintaining the integrity of the scenario in order to be able to highlight learning points for facilitators.

Bilingual simulated patients obviously require the same standard training in giving feedback as non-bilingual simulated patients. However, in addition to the basic training, you should remember to explore the problems of giving in-role feedback when the simulator has been portraying a character who speaks and understands no English.

There are basically three options for this:

➤ The simulated patient gives no in-role feedback and simply comes straight out of role at the end of the consultation. This is straightforward, but the benefits of direct in-role feedback are lost.

➤ The simulated patient gives in-role feedback in fluent English but maintaining the character of the role they have been portraying. This can be very difficult for some simulators to do, as the lack of comprehension is usually a major contributor to how they have been feeling.

➤ The simulated patient undergoes a 'virtual intensive language course' and so speaks and understands English but maintains an accent during feedback. This is only effective if the simulator has an accent naturally or is confident in assuming one.

The choices made here will need to be negotiated individually with the trainees, as any way of giving in-role feedback in these sessions is heavily reliant on the confidence of the simulated patient.

## Simulating health professionals

Ideally, a simulated patient would spend a period of time with a relevant health professional in order to fully assimilate important aspects of their working life. However, it is not generally possible to provide extensive additional training to enable people to simulate health professionals. It does, nevertheless, present quite a challenge to most simulated patients, and any measures you can take to equip them with relevant information about their supposed profession will help them to present as accurate a portrayal as is possible, without undertaking a 5-year medical degree or 20 years' experience as a ward sister!

Useful information may include:

➤ their professional duties and responsibilities

➤ their working conditions (e.g. shift patterns, hours)

➤ their attitudes (e.g. towards their work, their colleagues, health service policies)

➤ any professional (or unprofessional!) terminology or jargon they may use
    . . . actual words or phrases that they may use are particularly helpful.

## Simulating physical signs and symptoms

Using simulated patients to portray accurate physical signs and symptoms provides an extremely valuable resource for the teaching and assessment of clinical and diagnostic skills. However, if you would like your simulated patients to accurately portray physical signs and symptoms, whether for an assessment or for a teaching session, it is vital that they receive adequate training to do so in a convincing way. If a healthcare practitioner is intended to diagnose the problem from the signs and symptoms presented by the simulated patient, it is essential that the portrayal of these is completely accurate. Written instructions may occasionally be adequate for this, but it is far better if you can arrange for the simulated patient to spend some time with a practitioner in order to thoroughly understand the details of the problem.

For example, with a shoulder injury, the simulated patient should know the following:

➤ The type of pain they are experiencing and where precisely the pain is.
➤ Exactly when the pain occurs, whether it is on certain movements or whether it is continual (e.g. any limitations to movements as a result of the pain in, say, abduction, adduction or rotation). The simulated patient needs to know the precise movements and at which point the pain occurs.
➤ Whether there are any limitations to movements as a result of other causes (e.g. stiffness, blockage or weakness). The simulated patient needs to know the precise nature of the impediments.
➤ How they would respond to certain movements. Would they cry out in pain or just grimace slightly?
➤ Onset, radiation, associated symptoms, timescale, exacerbating and relieving factors, severity and any other aspects of history or effects on their daily life that they would need to know for most standard scenarios.

Training therefore, for simulating physical signs and symptoms should be very thorough and precise, and will benefit from the input of a specialist clinician.

You may wish to consider training specialist teams to portray a variety of physical signs and symptoms. One group of simulated patients may become experts in portraying knee conditions, for example, while another may specialise in cardiac problems. This allows them to focus on gaining a more in-depth understanding of certain areas of anatomy and physiology, allowing them to portray related problems with greater accuracy.

Another option for gaining this level of expertise is to use simulated patients who have existing or previous medical conditions. This enables a portrayal of a given role but can also include an authentic demonstration of physical signs and symptoms. You will obviously be limited to the medical conditions that have been experienced within your simulated patient resource, but it may allow for an authentic portrayal of physical signs and symptoms.

It is surprising how many physical conditions can be effectively simulated with high-level training, stage make-up and the cooperation of a skilled simulated patient! The potential for using simulated patients in these ways is increasingly being explored as it allows for more effective integration of clinical and interpersonal skills training.

### Assessment situations

If you wish to use simulated patients for an examination or high-level recruitment session, you should generally offer them extra training. This is to ensure consistency, an appropriate level of characterisation and a suitable pace of information giving. It is often a requirement of boards of assessment.

There are several crucial elements that you should cover in any additional training you offer to standardised patients.

### Focus

Explain to the simulated patients that the focus in an assessment situation is on providing a forum for the candidate to demonstrate their skills and knowledge. While, as ever, the simulated patients are required to present a convincing character, the focus in an examination is not to challenge and develop consultation techniques so much as to provide the candidates with a realistic setting whereby they may demonstrate the knowledge and skills they have already acquired.

### Consistency

Emphasise to the simulated patients that consistency is crucial. The examination situation differs from the training situation in that it is vital that the standardised patient maintains consistency in their portrayal of the role and in the giving of information. All candidates must be given an equal chance to demonstrate their knowledge and skill.

You can give them a useful tip to help achieve this: by using the same opening statement for each candidate, the standardised patient can, at least, give a consistent beginning to each encounter. From this point in, they will be reacting to how the candidate treats them, but at least each one will have been offered a fair start. Good examination training will make all the simulated patients who are performing the same scenario begin with the same opening statement.

Good assessment training will also try to ensure consistency in the delivery of the opening line. For example, if the first words are to be

'Well, I'm here with this cough again . . . it's not got any better.'

it is important to realise that these same words can be said in a depressed tone, an anxious tone or with frustration. Different intonation will express different emotions and therefore not present a standardised opening to each consultation. At a training session, it may be worth clarifying which emotion is intended to be conveyed and asking trainees to practise saying the opening line, in order to achieve consistency in emotion as well as in the actual words.

### Standardisation

You should ensure standardisation between simulated patients. If more than one standardised patient is going to be playing any one role, it is essential that they have the chance to meet together in order to standardise as much as possible the way they are portraying the character. Any clinical or social facts not specified within the brief should be developed with the help of a practitioner and should be the same for each station. Equally, there should be agreement about the intensity of emotion displayed by each standardised patient. If a patient is frustrated, it is essential that all simulators demonstrate a comparable level of frustration. It is not fair if one candidate faces a patient who is shouting at them because of the delay in their appointment while another patient merely mentions it and tuts.

At a training session, it may be worth spending some time exploring the different ways emotions can be portrayed and look at the physical manifestations of each. For example, frustration can be indicated by a movement of the lips or by banging a clenched fist on the table; for standardisation reasons, agreement should be reached in training as to which is the most appropriate. A list of physical indicators may be found in Appendix 4.

### Stamina

Warn the standardised patients that they may need great stamina in order to give everyone a fair chance. They may be required to do the same scenario many times in a single day (72 is my record but I am sure there are other simulated patients who could top that!). The simulator must present each candidate with the same starting point as the one before, whether they have just had some advice on giving up smoking or whether they have just been told they only have a short while to live. They must remember which pieces of information they have given to which candidate. They must be as focused and attentive at the end of the day as they were at the beginning.

### Facts

Point out how important it is that the standardised patients learn all clinical and social facts thoroughly, in order to recall them accurately. When given their scenario brief, it is absolutely crucial that the standardised patients learn all the clinical and social facts given. Remind them that the details in an examination scenario are carefully written to give the candidate the opportunity to demonstrate to the examiner his or her clinical knowledge and expertise. The examiner will have a marking sheet that corresponds to the factual knowledge that the simulators have in their scenario brief. Therefore, it is very important the standardised patients learn the correct information that they need to present to each candidate in response to their questioning.

### Sticking to the brief

Make it clear that the standardised patients must stick to the brief that they have been given.

It is essential that they do not alter their brief in any way – specifically, in any way that may have relevance to the outcome of the station. They may need to 'flesh out' the role, but they should exercise great caution in doing this and they should check any details they may wish to add with their examiner before the start. Certain social details may add realism without affecting the clinical outcome, but the simulator could inadvertently change the focus of the station with carelessly given answers.

For example, if the patient is seeing the doctor for chest problems and the standardised patient casually announces that they work in a sawmill, this could lead the candidate down a different and possibly incorrect path.

If the standardised patient is asked any clinical questions to which the answer was not in the scenario brief, you should tell them to answer in the negative. For example:

*Candidate:* 'Have you ever had anything like this before?'
*Standardised patient:* 'No, I don't think I've ever had anything like this before.'

Or:

*Candidate:* 'Do any heart conditions run in your family?'
*Standardised patient:* 'No, not that I know of.'

This is important, because if they invent a family history of, for example, heart disease, the candidate may pursue that line of questioning, when the character actually suffers from indigestion.

In the unlikely event, that the standardised patients are asked a clinical question to which they cannot remember the answer (unlikely because, of course, they will have learnt their scenario brief thoroughly!), suggest that they should try to be as vague and non-committal as possible. For example:

*Candidate:* 'How long have you been getting these headaches?'
*Standardised patient:* 'Well, it's hard to say really . . . hard to say when they actually started . . .'

It is better to be vague, as long as they can do it in a natural way, than to give potentially misleading information.

As well as needing to stick to clinical facts, it is also important that the standardised patients do not bring other emotions into the scenario. Obviously, as they are reacting, in some way, to the candidate's approach, they will show different emotions as a response. They may, for example, show relief if they feel reassured, or confusion if they do not understand something the candidate has said. This is ongoing feedback. However, ask them to avoid, for example, expressing strong emotions such as fear at the possible diagnosis, unless it is clearly mentioned in the scenario brief. Again, this may inadvertently lead the candidate away from the main issues and leave them short of time to cover the points that they are to be assessed on.

### Chunking

Crucially, you must teach the standardised patients to 'chunk' the information they give to the candidates. You need to talk about the importance of giving information in a controlled way, in order to give the practitioner a chance to demonstrate their skills. This is always important, but crucially so if you are training simulated patients for assessment purposes.

You may choose to demonstrate (or simply describe, depending on your resource availability) a short interaction:

*Practitioner:*   'Good morning. Can I just check . . . is it Irene Jenkins?'
*Simulated patient:*   'Yes, that's right.'
*Practitioner:*   'And how would you like me to address you?'
*Simulated patient:*   'Oh, Irene's fine.'
*Practitioner:*   'OK then, Irene, so what have you come to see the doctor about today?'
*Simulated patient:*   'Well, I've been getting these terrible pains in my stomach . . . awful they are. Real griping pains, almost every time I have anything much to eat, that's me . . . off to the loo, terrible tummy ache. I've had it ever since I was on holiday . . . I think it's something I've picked up over there . . . started as soon as we got off the plane last week and it's been getting worse ever since. I just hope it's not cancer . . . my father died of stomach cancer . . .'

Now tell the trainee simulated patients that the examiner has marks to allocate for the candidate who:
➤ introduces themselves appropriately
➤ asks about the nature of the problem
➤ asks how long it has lasted
➤ asks what the pains are like
➤ asks how frequently they occur
➤ asks whether anything in particular brings them on
➤ asks about family history
➤ asks if the patient has any ideas or concerns about the pain.

Ask the trainee simulated patients how many of those questions the practitioner would have been able to demonstrate. This should illustrate the point that if the standardised patient gives all the information about the condition in response to one question, then the examiner will not be able to assess whether or not the candidate knows which questions they need to ask and how to ask them appropriately.

### Methods of eliciting information
You should also talk about the various methods by which practitioners will try to elicit information. The simulated patients should be aware of the difference, for example, between open and closed questions and that deciding how much and what information to disclose in response is a challenge.

While no one expects the simulator to be deliberately evasive in any way, equally they should not offer information without feeling that the candidate has actually asked for it. The candidates need to be able to demonstrate to the examiner that they know which questions to ask and how to ask them. However, it is not that simple! In fact, this is probably one of the most difficult tasks for the standardised patient. Different candidates will obviously ask for information in different ways, and the patient must make continual judgements about how much and what information should be given in response.

It is not the case that unless a candidate uses specific words the standardised patient should not impart the information. If the candidate demonstrates appropriate skills, including the use of sensitively worded open questions and encouraging body language, the simulator should be more forthcoming, as a patient treated sensitively within a real consultation would undoubtedly be.

Ask the simulated patients to consider the following interaction:

*Candidate 1:*   'So, how long have you had this?'
*Standardised patient:*   'Oh, it must be about 3 or 4 weeks now?'
*Candidate 1:*   'And has it been getting any worse?'
*Standardised patient:*   'Well, no, not really ... but it's not getting any better either.'
*Candidate 1:*   'What is the pain like? Is it a sharp pain or a dull ache ...'
*Standardised patient:*   '... Well, it's more of a dull ache I suppose ...'
*Candidate 1:*   'Does it wake you up at night?'
*Standardised patient:*   'Well, yes, it does actually ...'
*Candidate 1:*   'And what about work? Does it stop you working?'
*Standardised patient:*   'Well, you just have to keep going really, don't you ...'

Ask them to consider the following interaction also:

*Candidate 2:*   'Can you tell me about this pain?'
*Standardised patient:*   'Well, it's a dull ache, sort of goes all around the back of my head ...'
*Candidate 2:*   '... uhuh ...?'
*Standardised patient:*   'Sometimes they're so bad, I just have to lie down ...'
*Candidate 2:*   (nods but stays quiet)
*Standardised patient:*   'I'm getting them most evenings now ...'
*Candidate 2:*   '... most evenings ...?'
*Standardised patient:*   'Yeah, almost every night I would say now ... I mean, they didn't use to be this often ... I'm sure they're getting worse ...
*Candidate 2:*   'It sounds like they're beginning to get you down?'
*Standardised patient:*   Yeah, well I'm just a bit worried, you know ...'

These are just brief snippets to illustrate how different the responses to the same station can be, and how difficult it is for the standardised patient to decide how much information to give in response to different questioning styles. In the first example we see that the candidate asked closed, focused questions. It is easier for the standardised patient to respond, given, as already seen, that they should try not to give information that has not been actually asked for. However, in the second example the candidate demonstrates effective consultation skills by asking open questions and using active listening skills (*see* Appendix 1). It is important that the standardised patient rewards the candidate for this and responds appropriately.

Sometimes the standardised patient brief includes specific guidance about what information should be given in response to effective open questioning and screening, and what information should really only be given if specifically asked for. This guidance is increasingly given in the standardised patient briefs, as examiners realise that if candidates display the consultation techniques being taught, then it is only fair to reward them appropriately. If the brief fails to include clear guidance as to the simulator's required responses, they will need to make their own judgements during the consultation.

The skill in deciding whether or not a piece of information has been asked for in an appropriately specific manner is one that the simulated patients will develop with experience. It is worth encouraging them to ask the assessor after the first station (if there is time) whether or not they provided a situation that enabled the examiner to effectively assess the candidate. If there is time between candidates, it is always worth the standardised patient checking with the examiner that they have played the role and responded to the interview appropriately.

### Confidence in signs and symptoms

Ensure the standardised patients are confident in how to portray any necessary physical signs and symptoms. If you require your simulated patients to portray physical signs and symptoms for diagnostic reasons, you must ensure that they all have a thorough knowledge of how to do this accurately.

It is important in an assessment situation that the knowledge the simulated patient has will allow for the demonstration of less-than-perfect examination techniques. For example, the simulator should know the extent and severity of the pain on pressure, or the effect of the full range of movements, and not just in response to an absolutely correct examination technique.

### Understanding the marking criteria

Ensure the standardised patients understand the marking criteria if they are to be involved with the actual assessment process. If the standardised patients are going to be assessing the candidates in any way, they will need to participate in a calibration exercise, in the same way that examiners do. It is important that all assessors, whether they be clinicians or standardised patients, use the same criteria for marking the candidates.

The most effective method of calibration is through videoing the consultation, which is then marked by the simulated patients. Their marks are compared and discussed, and any relevant guidance may be given to ensure consistency between them, in their approach to the candidates.

### Variations in process

You may need to give additional guidance on any specific variations in process. This may be as simple as indicating, for example, whether or not you wish the standardised patient to stay in the room at the end of each station. It may equally concern the simulated patient's role in the examination. If the assessment process involves the giving of some feedback, for example, you must indicate how proactive you would like the role of the simulated patient to be, or if you would like their feedback to be given in a particular way.

### Emotions

Make it clear to the standardised patients exactly how long emotional reactions should be sustained for. Ensure the standardised patients know that they are there to provide a forum for the candidates to demonstrate their knowledge and skills, rather than to recreate reality.

Depending on the level of the assessment, you may want the patient to sustain emotions that arise in a completely realistic way, even walking out if they feel that is what the patient would do. However, it is more likely that, for example, you will want the candidate to display a variety of skills, of which managing a patient's emotions is only one element. In this case, if a candidate says something that upsets the patient, the simulator should make this evident through ongoing feedback, thus giving them a chance to rectify the situation. However, it is then important that the simulator moves on and gives the candidate the chance to demonstrate the aspects of the consultation which they can perform better. For example, if a candidate introduces himself or herself poorly, it is important that the standardised patient responds to that for a short while but that they do not remain affronted or antagonistic for long, as this would affect the rest of the station. There may only be one mark for the introduction, but if the candidate is then dealing with an irritable person for the rest of the consultation, it may affect their overall performance, which may have been quite acceptable otherwise.

During the training process, the easiest way to make clear the important messages regarding the portrayal of the role and the giving of information is through demonstration. If possible, you could demonstrate a number of different 'candidates' (played by a simulated patient/facilitator) who could present a variety of challenges, as well as different portrayals of the same role by a simulated patient. For example, they may portray a student who asks completely closed questions and then one who uses active listening skills and open questioning. They may then demonstrate the pitfalls of giving too much information, not sticking to the information in the brief or becoming too focused on acting the role rather than on providing a forum for the candidate to demonstrate skills. Let the demonstrations run and then ask the group of trainee simulated patients to identify the features of each and why they may be problematic in an assessment situation. In this way, the messages you are trying to convey should be more clearly and firmly received.

# CHAPTER 5

# Writing scenarios and briefs

*You cannot dream yourself into a character; you must hammer and forge yourself one.*

Henry David Thoreau (1817–1862)

Unless you are using an agency (agencies can usually provide scenarios), or you have access to scenarios that your organisation has used before, you will find yourself in the position of needing to write your own.

Writing scenarios may at first seem relatively straightforward – indeed, it can be. However, there are some pitfalls to avoid, and by ensuring that the information given is as comprehensive as possible, you will improve the ease with which the learning outcomes can be achieved.

## WHO SHOULD WRITE SCENARIOS?

Both clinicians and non-clinical simulated patients or facilitators can write scenarios. The ideal situation is to have a small team or partnership that includes both, but this is rarely financially feasible. Therefore, it is important that all aspects are considered.

If you are a non-clinician writing a scenario, it is crucial that you have any clinical information that you wish to include checked by a clinician. The reason for this should be self-evident. Equally, if you are a clinical expert writing a scenario, it can also be extremely useful to have it checked by a simulated patient. It is amazing how much crucial information you can omit simply because you are used to approaching cases from a clinical perspective and have become so familiar with procedures or terminology that you assume a universal understanding.

> I was once helping a group of general practitioners to write some examination scenarios. I asked whether a patient with a particular condition would be taking medication. One of the doctors replied: 'We don't need to put that in. He probably wouldn't know . . . patients often don't know what medication they are taking.'
>
> Even if patients don't remember the name of the medication they are

taking, they usually tend to know whether or not they are taking something, and whether it is a couple of white tablets or a spoonful of medicine that they are swallowing! Therefore, at the very least, the simulated patient needs to know this.

When writing, you should always bear in mind the information that you are hoping the practitioner will elicit and include it in your scenario. This sounds obvious but, believe me, it doesn't always happen! You need to think about the ideal outcome for the scenario and provide all the information relevant for this; however, you also need to consider which other paths the practitioner may explore in order to reach that outcome, and provide that information for the simulated patient. This may also need to include 'negatives', or those symptoms which the patient doesn't have, as well as those they do.

Some information may not appear relevant to a scenario, but you should always prepare your simulated patient for the unexpected! For example, a less confident practitioner will often fall back on unnecessary checklists to compensate for a lack of knowledge. If the simulated patient doesn't have the necessary information to deal with this, this can affect their confidence and their portrayal of the role. You may also run the risk of the simulated patient inventing inappropriate information and inadvertently sidetracking the consultation.

Although some background information may appear unimportant, it can still be very useful for the simulated patient to understand more about the character they are playing. It can give the simulated patient more confidence in their responses if they are sure of the information they are giving.

I have devised the following template to help you write a comprehensive scenario. Clearly, not all the information will be relevant to every situation. However, it will be useful to consider each section and make a thoughtful decision about which information to include.

If you decide that an aspect of social history really is unimportant, make it clear in the scenario that the simulated patient can create this information for themselves.

## SCENARIO WRITING TEMPLATE
### Learning points
First of all and for purposes of maintaining focus, you may want to identify the learning points you are aiming for in the scenario. These may include some of the following or different ones according to the needs of the group.

**Medical** – including learning points around any actual health problems and treatment options.
**Psychological** – including the psychological impact of these health problems on the person's life, as well as any underlying psychological issues.
**Social** – encouraging a holistic view of the person's life and appreciating the importance of the issue of social support.

**Communication** – including communication both within the interaction and beyond, written and verbal.

**Ethical** – including any ethical issues that may affect the situation.

**Teamwork** – communicating with other members of the healthcare team, making referrals, other support.

**Health promotion** – learning how to make use of ad hoc health promotion opportunities.

**Professional integrity** – exploring issues about professional integrity that may arise within this scenario.

You may wish to do this exercise simply to maintain your own focus, or you may choose to share the learning points with other facilitators, with the simulated patients or even with the group, depending on the objectives of the session and the maturity of the group.

### Factual information

You will then need to give all the factual details of the scenario. You should ensure that all necessary information is given. If you decide that any details can be left for the simulated patient to generate, you should specify this in the scenario.

### Name

Choose a name or specify that the simulated patient can choose their own. If you choose the name, be aware of any cultural implications that the name may have.

### Age range

Remember the wider the age range is, the easier it is to find suitable simulated patients.

### Gender

Again, if the scenario can be interchangeable, then it gives more scope for recruiting good simulated patients.

### Ethnicity

Give the ethnicity of the patient if this is relevant to the scenario; otherwise, specify that ethnicity choice can be any.

### Setting of interaction

Where does the interaction itself take place (e.g. in the waiting room, in outpatients, in the person's home and so forth)?

### Reason for interaction

Why has the patient come to see the doctor/health practitioner? What is the primary purpose of the interaction? Why have they come to see the practitioner at this particular time?

### Background

What is the background to the presenting problem? This is where you can indulge your penchant for the acronym and the tick box! Students and practitioners often learn to use them, so there is every chance the questions will be asked. It is helpful therefore, to equip your simulated patient with the answers!

The most useful is the acronym for eliciting a history of pain, which can be adapted and used more generally within a consultation: SOCRATES (Site, Onset, Character, Radiation, Associated symptoms, Time course, Exacerbating/alleviating factors, Severity – say, on a scale of 0–10).

Other common tick box lists and acronyms are more specific to particular scenarios and include the following.

➤ Depression scenarios: sleep pattern, concentration, appetite, mood, enjoyment of life, intention of self-harm.
➤ Addiction scenarios: CAGE (have you ever felt you should Cut down on drinking? Do you feel Annoyed when others criticise your drinking? Do you ever feel Guilty about your drinking? Have you ever needed an Eye-opener in the morning?).
➤ Other mental health scenarios: ASEPTIC (Appearance and behaviour; Speech; Emotion – mood and affect; Perception – hallucination and illusion; Thought content and process; Insight and judgement; Cognition).

You should also note the absence of symptoms that could mislead the practitioner.

### Social history

It is useful to include here family situation, employment status and other relevant social factors. You may mention how the person feels about their current social circumstances, if it is relevant to the scenario.

When choosing social details, always consider potential implications; for example, if you have a patient with breathing difficulties, if they worked as a stonemason their situation would be very different to if they were working in an office. Such details may also have an impact on the differential diagnoses and management options offered by the practitioner.

### Lifestyle

This includes information about the person's diet, alcohol intake, smoking, exercise and other lifestyle factors. Again, be careful that you don't inadvertently take the consultation down the wrong path by making your patient drink too much, for example.

### Past medical history

Has the person had any previous illnesses and operations? If there is nothing significant, you should note this; otherwise, an inexperienced simulated patient may think they are to create this themselves.

### Family history

Have any members of the patient's family had any relevant illnesses or diseases? Again, mention if there is nothing significant.

### Medication

What medication is a patient taking? Include both prescribed and over-the-counter medications. Here it is helpful to give the medical names as well as how the patient might describe them (e.g. diuretics, a specific drug name, water tablets, little white tablets and so forth). Include also any complementary healthcare treatments.

### Allergies

Is there anything that the person is allergic to? What happens to them when they have an allergic reaction?

### Patient's perspective

This is where you can describe the patient's temperament and feelings, both generally, and about the current situation. It is as important to be as thorough in this section as in the more factual section, as these are the details that both create the personality of the character and furnish the simulated patient with information vital to the practitioner in order to effectively manage the situation.

### Temperament

How would you describe the patient's basic personality? For example, are they phlegmatic or irascible? Are they extrovert or shy? How have they responded to recent events?

### Ideas

What does the patient believe is causing the problem? You should also indicate where they got those ideas from; for example, did they know someone with similar symptoms, did they look on the Internet, did they read a magazine?

### Concerns

What is the patient most worried about? These concerns may be directly related to the situation. They may also include less obvious anxieties, which patients often worry about more than the immediate problem.

### Expectations

What does the patient want from this consultation, what do they expect and what would their ideal outcome be? You may also indicate how entrenched these expectations are and how they would feel if these expectations were not met. You may need to suggest how the simulated patient should react to a selection of possible options that may be offered to them.

### Behaviour

This is a very important section as it gives the simulated patient guidance on how to conduct themselves during the consultation. This should include how you would like the patient to begin the consultation (possibly including an opening statement). You should identify the person's general mood, and if, how much and under what circumstances this should change during the consultation. You should give indications of any reactions required for specific questions, comments and so forth. You may also want to give examples of comments that the patient may make to convey certain points.

You could indicate what level and type of challenge you would like the simulated patient to offer. Often consultations are not challenging because of their medical learning points, but because of a difficulty in interacting with the patient. This is the section where you can indicate the levels and types of challenge you feel would be helpful for a particular group or individual. If, for example, you are writing a scenario for 'breaking bad news', do you want the person to be overtly upset or shocked? If you are writing a scenario for a workshop on managing conflict, do you want the simulated patient to be irritated, angry or aggressive? If they are angry, is this a quiet fury or do you want loud verbal abuse?

You may also wish to indicate reactions to specific interventions. For example, if you are writing a scenario describing a timid, unassertive patient, you may wish to indicate what strategies employed by the practitioner may encourage them to speak.

### Impact on life

You may wish to suggest ways in which the problems the patient is facing are affecting his/her daily life. You should indicate these in order of their severity.

### Feelings

You may suggest any additional feelings the patient may have that have not been mentioned in any of the previous categories.

### Variations

You may wish to suggest ways of varying the role in order to present different challenges. These could be factual changes or variations in the patient's perspective, personality or behaviour.

### Timeline

A timeline can be very useful, especially when the case has a complex history.

### Opening statement

This is a very important aid for achieving consistency. If the simulated patient begins each consultation with each candidate with the same words, said in the same way, at least each candidate is then presented with the same opening chance.

It is also invaluable in promoting consistency between simulated patients if you have more than one doing any one station. The manner in which the opening line is said can be practised at a training session, but even with slight discrepancies between simulated patients, at least each candidate is hearing the same words.

### Writing other briefs

You may also need to write a practitioner's brief. This sets the scene for the person or people carrying out the consultation. This doesn't need to be long but can clarify the following points.

#### Setting

Where does the interaction take place? Is this the practitioner's normal place of work? Are there any other specific details about the setting that may have an impact on how the consultation is managed?

#### Reason for the interaction

What knowledge do they have about why the patient wants to speak to them? Is the interaction to be initiated by the patient or by the practitioner?

#### Practitioner's role

What is the practitioner's role within this setting? Do they have any specific tasks to carry out within the consultation?

#### Additional clinical information

Sometimes it is helpful to provide information that the practitioner may need to carry out a task within the consultation.

#### Additional social factors

For example, how well does the practitioner know the patient? How is the practitioner's own personal situation? Are there additional stresses inherent in the setting or the task?

Always bear the learning objectives for the session in mind when writing the practitioner's brief. For example, if the aim is to practise the giving of information rather than the taking of the history, you may choose to give more information in the practitioner's brief. If the aim is managing conflict, you may give no information.

Sometimes medical notes should be given to create a realistic background for the consultation and to give necessary information about the person's past medical history.

If you are working with other facilitators, you may need to write a facilitator's brief. It is important that you are all aware of the learning aims of the session and the essential details of the process.

## Writing examination scenarios

You can use the same template for writing examination stations as for writing teaching scenarios. However, it is even more important that you are clear and precise with your information. If there is ambiguity within a teaching session and the session goes awry, the facilitator can simply stop it and set it back on its anticipated course. However, if there are unaddressed anomalies within the scenario for an examination, and a candidate is misled as a result, there is usually less scope for rectifying the situation.

As all simulated patients should have a training session before any major examinations in order to calibrate the roles, it would be hoped that any ambiguities would be identified and rectified before the examination. However, if you can try to be as clear as possible when writing the scenarios in the first place, it ultimately saves time, effort and possible disaster!

When writing examination scenarios, it is crucial to match up the information given to the simulated patient with the skills you wish to elicit from the candidate. The writing of the scenario and the marking scheme must go hand in hand. You should check every detail of the scenario with the marking scheme to ensure that it allows for the desired outcomes to be reached by the successful candidate. If possible, you should try to incorporate some information within the scenario that will act as a differentiator between competent and incompetent candidates, but again you should make sure that this differentiation is reflected in the marking scheme.

It is also important to try to practise an examination scenario. Often, when creating a scenario, you can imagine how it may unfold in the examination, but you may find that in practice the unexpected is far more common! The theoretical outcomes are often not matched by the actual outcomes, and it is essential that adequate testing of the scenario identifies any potential difficulties in the scenario before it is actually used in an assessment situation.

> I was once working with a group of consultants, writing a series of examination stations for a medical school OSCE [objective structured clinical examination]. Once we had developed the scenarios and established the marking schemes for the stations, we decided to practise them. Each scenario was attempted by all eight senior doctors to ensure the viability of the station. Six out of the eight consultants who tried one of the more straightforward stations failed it! This could be a very worrying indicator of a lack of expertise within the medical profession, but it was actually more a reflection of how important it is to make sure the marking scheme corresponds to the written scenario. It is amazing how many changes usually need to be made to marking schemes and scenarios after practice!

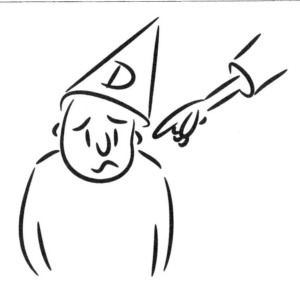

**'Must try harder!'**

### Writing forum scenarios

The use of forum theatre is described in more detail in Chapter 9. The following are some guidelines on writing a forum scenario and the preparation for such a session, but it is recommended that you read these in conjunction with the section on forum theatre.

If you are using a forum theatre presentation to explore communication issues, you still need to give a full scenario brief to each simulated patient. As they will need to remain in role for a sustained period of time, it is very important that they are confident in the character they are portraying.

If, as is likely in a forum theatre situation, some or all of your simulators are playing the parts of professionals, you will need to give them some guidance on this (*see* Chapter 4). In addition to the comprehensive scenarios that are given to each character, you will need to decide how you would like to present the initial interaction.

You may decide to write a short script involving each character. This could, for example, follow the build-up of a tense situation ending in overt conflict or it could simply highlight a difficult situation.

Alternatively, you may choose to write a detailed brief of the anticipated action, so that you are giving guidance for how the characters are to interact and how the conflict will be built up. However, you will not be providing an exact script for the simulated patients to learn verbatim. Instead, they will improvise within the guidelines of the brief.

There should be a clear indication within the script or detailed brief regarding when the facilitator would stop the action and begin the next phase of the session. You could decide to write a 'cue' line to be spoken by one of the characters, or you could simply indicate that when emotions reached a certain pitch then the facilitator should stop the action.

After the initial presentation, the group will be directing the action themselves. The simulated patients will be working from the information they learnt from the original scenario brief and from the instructions given them by their groups.

## PART THREE

# Managing the session

*It turns out that an eerie type of chaos can lurk just behind a facade of order – and yet, deep inside the chaos lurks an even eerier type of order.*

Douglas Hofstadter (b. 1945)

# CHAPTER 6

# Immediate preparation

## ENVIRONMENTAL REQUIREMENTS FOR SESSION

Your input into the actual booking of a venue and provision of facilities will depend largely on the type of session you are running and on the type of organisation you are working for. It may be that rooms are allocated within the institution for which you are working or it may be that you have to organise this yourself.

If you have rooms already allocated, you should endeavour to visit the rooms before the start of the session, in order to make sure they are suitable for your needs. You may have to change the layout of the furniture or ask for additional equipment.

If you have responsibility for organising the venue and environment, you need to consider how best to go about this. Whether you have decided to book your simulated patients through an agency or to recruit independently, you will first need to identify the environmental requirements for your session. If you are using an agency, it is often possible for them to arrange a venue and provide equipment; however, you will still need to specify exactly what you need.

Whether you have the budget to book a prestigious hotel for your workshop, decide to use teaching rooms in your local hospital or use the reception area of a general practice surgery, you should bear in mind the following points.

### Venue

➤ Does the venue have the capacity for your group?
➤ Is it accessible to all?
➤ Is there a room large enough for whole group activities, such as an introductory warm-up and plenary? If you are running a forum theatre session, you need a room whereby an audience can view a 'performance' but with the possibility of splitting into smaller groups within the same room.
➤ Are there breakout rooms for small-group work? For example, you may be using three simulated patients who will go to three groups in sequence. It is better, if possible, to have three small rooms rather than one large one.

➤ If there is only a large room available, is it possible to divide the room in any way? If so, will it be sufficient for the types of scenario you are using, or might you need to adjust the scenarios slightly? It can be quite disconcerting for all concerned, trying to discuss the intricacies of bowel movements to a backing track of inconsolable sobbing or threats of violence! If your physical resources enforce close proximity between simultaneous scenarios, it is better to ask the simulated patient to temper the expression of high emotions.

## Equipment

You need to consider whether or not you will need such equipment as PowerPoint facilities, flip charts, paper and pens to be provided for the group. Also, if it is a group you do not know, consider whether or not they should be given name badges to ease initial communication. If you are running a telephone consultation session, you may need to ensure the phone equipment is working in the way you want it to.

> I was quite shocked to notice, on the paperwork for an examination station, the following.
>
> Equipment requirements:
> - One blood pressure monitor
> - One timer
> - One simulated patient.
>
> Still, as I mentioned in the Introduction, simulated patients do have to get used to being called a variety of names . . . a piece of equipment is probably not the worst!

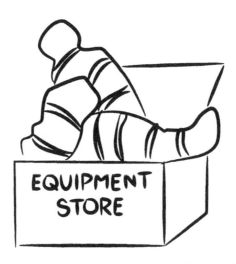

**'I hope none of these got damaged in transit!'**

## Seating arrangements

You should think about the seating arrangements. Desks are rarely useful; the most common arrangement is a horseshoe of chairs enabling people to watch the enactment of a consultation. A larger group forum session may be better organised into small groups, as they watch the forum theatre presentation, so that they are ready for the separate group discussion afterwards.

## Catering

➤ Will you be offering refreshments?
➤ Does the venue have catering facilities? If not, how will you provide refreshments?
➤ What refreshments do you need to order or have the budget for?
➤ If you have a limited budget for refreshments, is it clear to the participants and the simulated patients exactly what will be provided?
➤ If the participants and/or the simulated patients are expected to provide their own refreshments, do they know what facilities are available, if any, on-site?

## Scene setting

It is sometimes useful to think about how much physical scene setting would be useful. This can vary from two chairs in a room to some forum sessions that may resemble an amateur dramatics performance with full props and lighting.

Usually you will provide an environment somewhere between these two. If a person is supposed to be lying in a hospital bed, it is useful, for example, to have access to a suitable piece of furniture for the simulated patient to lie on, as this physical situation has an impact on the communication, and there may be

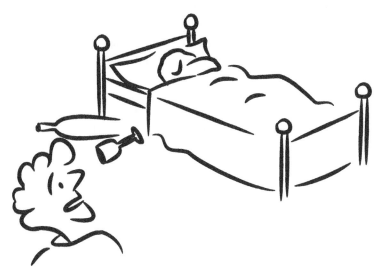

'Good morning Mr Granger . . .'

some learning points to be drawn from this. Similarly, if a home visit is to be simulated, then a few props may help to create some realism to help illustrate some of the learning points. You will need to think about who will provide any props or equipment you may use. What can the venue provide? Do you need to bring anything or ask the simulated patients to bring anything?

> One home visit scenario I was once working on required the simulated patient couple to be living in squalor. The use of beer cans, half-eaten takeaway food, broken toys, cigarette ends and a blaring radio, which, on request, was only slightly turned down, really helped illustrate some of the difficulties inherent in such an interaction.
>
> It wasn't much fun clearing up afterwards though!

## AIMS AND OBJECTIVES

When you are considering the aims and objectives of your session, you must first ascertain how strongly tied you are to the aims of the organisation within which you are working. If there are pre-established learning outcomes, you should find out whether or not you are allowed any flexibility within these. This session may be an integral part of a syllabus or a training programme, in which case you may, for example, have to make history taking your main focus.

It is useful to clearly work out your aims and objectives beforehand, as it is helpful to explain the raison d'être of the session to the group. It may be a part of the core curriculum at a healthcare training institution. It may be that there has been a customer satisfaction survey at the surgery and this is a way of addressing some of the issues arising from this. Perhaps some funding has become available and it has been felt that the ancillary staff of a hospice have long been overlooked in training provision. Whatever prompted the session however, it should always be presented as an opportunity for development rather than a corrective process, in order to engage the group in a positive way.

Even when you have fairly rigid learning outcomes to work towards, it is still useful to identify any specific ideas from the group, about what they would like to get from the session. It is usually possible to incorporate additional objectives into a simulated patient session, since by its very nature it is a flexible medium. You will find the group will be more engaged with the process if it is tailored to their own needs. The process of ascertaining the individual learning objectives of the group members can be, in itself, a useful warm-up exercise to help the group get to know each other and to focus on the task in hand.

# CHAPTER 7

# Dynamic groups or group dynamics

*A teacher who is attempting to teach without
inspiring the pupil with a desire to learn
is hammering on a cold iron.*

Horace Mann (1796–1859)

## GETTING THE GROUP ON BOARD!

### Assessing the group

It is important to make an informal assessment of your group before you begin the session, as you will need to adapt your material and methods accordingly. What may be very effective, in terms of process and scenario, with a group of dentists may not work so well with a group of accident and emergency nurses, and vice versa! An inter-professional learning group will present yet more challenges as well as additional opportunities for sharing best practice and developing team-working strategies.

Just as a practitioner should find out the ideas, concerns and expectations of a patient before they can effectively help them, so it will probably improve the outcomes of your group if you know what their idea of simulated patient work is, what they are most worried about and what they are hoping to get from it!

It is useful to ask yourself the following questions:

➤ How large is the group? You will need to know this during the early part of the planning stage of the session, as you need to employ very different strategies and techniques to get the best out of groups of varying sizes.

➤ How well do the group members know each other? It may be a group that has studied together for some time, for example, or it may be a group of work colleagues, with a variety of relationships within it, or it may be a group that has never met before.

➤ How well do you know the group, and how do you see yourself in relation to this group? You may be their employer, or tutor. You may be a complete stranger, invited in to run a series of workshops or a one-off session with them.

➤ Are they from the same discipline as one another and are they from the

same discipline as you are? If not, you need to make a decision as to whether you need to do any research into their background.
➤ Are they all at the same level of training? Do they have a similar amount of experience as one another?
➤ Do any of the group members have prior experience of working with simulated patients?

If anyone has previously worked with simulated patients, it is useful to find out how they felt about it – honestly! Some health professionals are very familiar with this way of working, while others may have limited or no experience whatsoever. For example, often professionals who have trained overseas will have no experience of consultation skills training. They may feel very anxious because they are not really sure what to expect and will need more reassurance and explanation. Equally, if anyone has had a damaging experience of working with simulated patients previously, it is worth making the effort to explore this so you can endeavour to improve it for them this time. The time spent doing this is usually worth it to highlight and begin to eliminate any potential antipathy towards the session.

Do you know of any overt difficulties within the group dynamics? This may be information you have been given or have experienced, or it may be information that you gain during the early part of the session/s. You may have a very assertive, confident practitioner who dominates all discussion, or a couple of very shy individuals who are reluctant to participate in any way.

What are the members of the group hoping to learn from the session? For example, have they come with a specific agenda of their own, or are they simply attending a compulsory staff training day that gives them a nice break from the daily routine but, beyond that, they haven't given it a second thought? The motivation and levels of enthusiasm for participating in this consultation session will have a huge impact on how the group engage with the process, and how much work you have to do to manage the situation.

All this information is useful as, for example, you may choose to use alternative scenarios with an inter-professional group of practitioners, or an alternative feedback model with a group comprising people with different levels of training and experience. Equally, the type and degree of feedback given would vary enormously depending on the basic attitude and confidence of the group and the professional backgrounds of the individuals, as well as the learning outcomes sought. We will look at this in more detail in Chapter 11.

You will also face a huge variation in the level of challenge you will face between a coerced group and a group of enthusiastic volunteers!

The experience of working with a group of motivated and thoughtful professionals who have chosen to come on a workshop in order to enhance their consultation skills can be such a positive, almost invigorating experience! Such sessions take on a life of their own and the facilitator can find it more of a shared learning journey than a teaching session.

At the other end of the scale, working with a group of medical students on a Friday morning (after the seemingly obligatory Thursday night out on the town) can leave a facilitator feeling as though they have been dowsed in treacle!

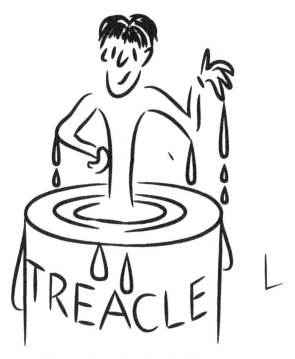

**The morning after the night before . . .**

Just as each person is an individual and every interaction is unique, so each group has its own dynamics and every simulated patient session presents a different challenge. It is your job as facilitator to continually assess the group. You need to use your skills, intuition and judgement to develop the most effective ways of using the simulated patient consultation to help each practitioner achieve their own learning outcomes.

### How do you assess the group?

There are different ways of making your judgements about the group, depending largely on the particular circumstances surrounding each session.

Some information you must have before the session, as the types of activities you decide to include will depend on your assessment of the group.

➤ You may be given or have acquired prior information about the group.
➤ You may have the opportunity to get to know the group as part of an ongoing training programme.
➤ You may be able to send out a pre-session questionnaire to find out the background, levels of experience, expectations and so forth of the group members. This has the added advantage of focusing the participants before

the session, and even enabling you to set tasks related to the session, to help the group members arrive more prepared for the challenges of the session. For example, you may ask them to identify a specific communication challenge they have encountered or witnessed in practice.

➤ If you have not had a chance to meet the group prior to the session, you should observe them from the outset. You are trying to identify, for example, friendship groupings, general attitudes and overt group dynamics. You may ask them about their experience, both clinically and of working with simulated patients.

You can be making this assessment as people arrive, and then carefully thought-out introductions and warm-ups can give you further opportunity.

While making your judgements about the group and decisions about how to tailor your session accordingly, you should be aware of your own prejudices. You may imagine you have a pretty good idea of, for example, 'typical orthopaedic surgeon' behaviour or 'typical practice receptionist' attitude, but it is important that you acknowledge this prejudice to yourself, and then try not to be closed to the individuality of the group members. You may be surprised!

### Setting off!

So, you have begun to make your assessment of the group. It is your job to get the best out of this session with this particular group of people, whether they are already buzzing with enthusiasm or slumped in their chairs with a glazed look in their eyes!

You should never scrimp on the time needed to get a new group warmed up! There are often a lot of issues that affect how people approach the challenge of working with simulated patients. The use of simulated patients is increasing all the time; however, although more and more people may have experience of this way of working, it doesn't necessarily mean that their experience was a good one, or that they feel they could benefit from another session. It could be that they were a victim of overcritical feedback from an inexperienced simulated patient during their nurse training and so are dreading the whole experience. It could be that they had some consultation skills training in their second year at medical school but now, in their third year, feel they do not need further training with 'pretend patients' as they are now practising taking histories from 'real patients' on the wards.

### Warm-ups

Different groups will need different warm-ups, both in quantity and in content. A selection of different exercises that may be useful with different groups of practitioners is provided here. This is by no means an exhaustive list and there are many resources available, and suggested for further reading, that give ideas for encouraging a group to become cohesive and effective.

I think it is very important that everybody in the room has spoken before the actual consultation part of the session begins. Obviously, the way in which this is achieved will depend on the size of the group and how well the participants already know one another.

If you are hoping people will volunteer to walk out to the front of the room to carry out a consultation at some point during the session, it can be useful to get the group members to move, in some way, during the warm-up. Most of these exercises can be further enhanced, especially with a larger group, by making everyone stand and move around the room. This may be to carry out tasks or simply to change places with someone else. If they have once broken out from the security of the chair they have initially made their comfort zone, then there is a greater chance they may do it again!

### Conversation

These can be simple and spontaneous conversations that involve yourself and the whole group. If it is a group you work with on a regular basis, you may ask how things have gone since you last met, both generally and, more specifically, whether they have encountered any challenging communication issues. If it is a new group, you may ask where they work, or how they're feeling about the prospect of working with simulated patients.

### Ground rules

Setting ground rules with the group can be a useful way of getting people to focus on the aims of the session and also can be used to encourage a feeling of safety and support within the group. You could divide them into pairs or small groups to discuss what principles about being in this group are important to them. The group can then come back together to write them on a flip chart as their established group rules.

### Defining learning outcomes

Defining or refining the learning outcomes people are hoping to achieve from the session/s can be another useful way of getting people to speak in the first instance; it also gives you an idea of the expectations of the group. You can do this in a number of different ways, from straight conversation within the large group or smaller groups through to some way of writing them down and then sharing them with others.

### Speaking in small groups

If practitioners seem reluctant to engage in a discussion within the whole group, it is useful to ask them to speak in pairs or groups of three about a specific point, and then they can share the outcome of their discussions with the rest of the group. This helps less confident practitioners to focus their ideas and it takes the pressure off them to speak spontaneously, in front of the whole group. It also helps to begin building relationships within the group.

### Discussing hopes and fears

Discussing 'hopes and fears' about the session at the beginning in pairs can provide a focus for establishing ground rules.

### Discussing session task

It can be useful to initiate a discussion based on the task of the session. For example, I often use the following activity if I am initiating a session on talking about difficult news.

Draw the following diagram on the board/flip chart:

| environment | practitioner | task | patient/relative/colleague |
|---|---|---|---|
|  |  |  |  |

Divide the group into four subgroups and give each group one of the areas. Then ask them to discuss what issues relating to their area they would want to consider before embarking on the interaction. Coming back to the main group, I would write their thoughts down on the board/flip chart and leave this in view during the consultation. This warm-up activity enables everyone to speak in a smaller, less intimidating group, and would focus everyone's thoughts on the task ahead.

### Introductions

If you have a new group, you will need to find a way to get the members to introduce themselves. You can simply go round and ask people to give their name and a little information about their background (or any other information you feel you would like them to share). However, a word of recommendation: if you are ever asking people to speak individually within the large group, don't go round the circle sequentially. This often has the result that half the group are not listening to what others are saying, as they are watching the moment approach when they will have to speak themselves. The effect of this is lessened if you are more random in the order in which you invite people to speak, though you must make sure you don't leave anyone out!

### Introduction to neighbour

You can make this exercise more interesting and less threatening if you ask them to introduce themselves to their neighbour, finding out from each other their relevant details and then introducing their neighbour to the rest of the group. This can be livelier and more fun (therefore more relaxing!) if you introduce another element into this task. You could ask them to find out their partner's name, professional background and, for example, something unusual about themselves, something they are proud of or something they hope to achieve in the next 10 years. The list is endless and is useful in introducing the group participants as human beings rather than simply as members of a certain profession.

### Introduction at a party
A development of this exercise is to ask them to walk around the room imagining they are at a party. For some sessions it may even be appropriate to have some background music as this is happening, to create more of an atmosphere. Then, on a given signal, they should stop and introduce themselves and maybe ask one question to another group member/partygoer. After a time for a short discussion, another signal indicates that they move, as a pair, until the next signal. This time, they meet another pair and perhaps answer and discuss a different question in a group of four, and so on. The questions can become ever more focused to the learning outcomes of the session. For example:

➤ In pairs you may ask them to introduce themselves and find out something interesting which their partner has done in the last year.
➤ Then, still in their pairs, they move on together and join another pair and, following introductions, they could find out what each other's biggest challenges were at work or with communication, for example.
➤ This can then be repeated with other pairs and different questions becoming ever more focused on the session.

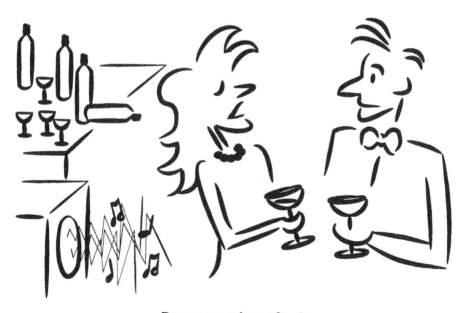

**Do you come here often?**

### Exploring verbal and non-verbal communication

Warm-ups that focus on exploring people's experience of communication may be useful to begin the process of exploring our verbal and non-verbal signals and responses.

Divide the group into pairs. One member of each pair then begins to describe, to their partner, an interest or a hobby which they feel absolutely passionate about, but they describe it in a totally impassionate way, as though the whole topic is completely boring to them.

After 2 minutes you allow them to express their interest in a way that reflects the enthusiasm they feel about the subject. After a further 2 minutes, swap roles and repeat the exercise.

Bring the group back together and discuss the experience. Discussion will usually highlight use of such things as eye contact, tone, volume, body language and hand gestures. It can then be used to relate communication indicators to mood and how certain communications affect a person's feelings.

### Highlighting communication issues

A similar exercise involves a series of interactions whereby responses to communication are limited. Again, dividing the group into pairs you can set them a variety of tasks; for example, they may sit back-to-back with each person talking in turn for 3 minutes on a subject that is important to them. The other person must simply listen and make no response.

They may then move to be face-to-face and repeat the exercise, with a different subject and the same or a different partner. This time the listener can only respond non-verbally.

The listener in each pair could then be asked to interrupt, clarify and comment on every single point made by the speaker. They may do the exercise with one person seated and the other standing, or even with one partner lying on the floor. Possibilities are endless and can be created to highlight different communication issues.

### Miming

If you are organising a session exploring difficulties in consulting with patients who have difficulty expressing themselves in English, you could try using the warm-up described in Chapter 4, which involves participants miming a complex problem or anxiety. This is a fun activity that begins to highlight some of the challenges in an interaction where the two people do not have a shared verbal language.

### Short forum presentation

You may decide to use a short forum presentation (*see* Chapter 9) as a warm-up before more intensive small-group work. If, for example, you have three simulated patients ready to work in three small groups, you could give them either a scripted or semi-scripted piece to perform at the beginning of the session. This could then be directed in a forum theatre way to explore some of the communication issues. This can be a very effective way of introducing a session, as it gives the practitioners in the group a chance to become involved in the situation in a completely non-threatening way. They should feel more confident, as they are directing the actors rather than being a part of the actual interaction. This enables them to move on to the smaller-group work, feeling validated in their capabilities as they have watched their suggestions played out on the stage earlier and therefore more willing to participate in the more intense, interactive work.

### Other ideas

There are a host of games and exercises that may be used as ice-breakers. They should always be short, and they should be carefully thought through to ensure that they create the required atmosphere for the session. It is important that you choose activities that are appropriate for the group participants so that they don't find them patronising or, indeed, threatening. Carefully chosen, however, they can help hugely in relaxing the group for the task in hand.

### Warmed up for what?! Setting the scene

So you have the group happily on board and ready to set off on this exciting voyage of discovery! Your next job is to make sure they know the approximate route you are hoping to take so that they can all play their part in keeping the session on course and achieve the hoped-for learning outcomes.

It is important that all group members are clear about the process in order for the session to run smoothly; although some things may become apparent during the course of the consultation, the more you can prepare the participants for the process, the more they can focus on the content.

You should already know what the experience of your group is with regard to working in this way. However, it is useful to emphasise that even if they have participated in simulated patient sessions previously, there are many different approaches that can be adopted. They may not all have worked in the exact way you are about to work. Everyone should be clear about the basic structure of this particular session and the nature of their contribution to it.

In particular, you should make the participants aware of the following points.
➤ The learning outcomes (negotiated and/or predetermined).
➤ The way the session will run.
➤ Whether the consultation is intended to run from start to finish with no interruptions.
➤ Whether you are allowing time out for discussion.
➤ Whether you are using different techniques such as hot-seating to gather information.
➤ How the session can be stopped.
➤ Who can ask for time out? I would always emphasise at this point that if I, as facilitator, decided to pause a session, it would not mean that the practitioner doing the consultation had done anything wrong, but simply

that I felt there may be value to be gained from some group discussion at this point. We will talk about why you may feel it appropriate to stop the session in Chapter 9. You should consider, before you start, which of these reasons it may be useful to share with the group at the beginning of the session.

➤ How the practitioners can pause for help.
➤ When the simulated patient will be in role or out of role and how the group will know.
➤ How feedback will be given.
➤ In what order feedback will be given.
➤ Who will manage the feedback.
➤ Whether you would like the practitioners to validate their observations with the simulated patient in role during discussions.
➤ Whether the simulated patient will give feedback in or out of role at the end.
➤ What kind of feedback you expect them to give (e.g. supportive, descriptive, constructive, specific and so forth).
➤ What you would like them to notice during the consultation.
➤ Whether you want them to give feedback on specific behaviours.
➤ Whether you want the interviewing practitioner to identify areas for feedback they would like to receive, before you begin.
➤ Whether you want the group to be taking notes during the consultation.
➤ What kind of things they should be noting down.
➤ Whether you want individual group members to have specific tasks.
➤ Any other aspects of the session they need to know (e.g. timings, other tasks and so forth).

### The willing volunteer

At last you are ready to focus on your first consultation! Obviously, you and the group will need to decide which practitioner is going to begin the first consultation. However much you have relaxed your group in preparation, the initial volunteer may not leap to their feet as soon as you have uttered the words 'Who would like to go first?' Much like a doctor discussing an embarrassing problem with a patient, the best approach is often to be (or at least to pretend to be) calm and matter-of-fact about the whole thing, and to use humour, as ever, to relax the situation.

Here are a few tactics you may wish to consider employing. First, you can simply choose a practitioner to begin the consultation. Sometimes this is inevitable, but if you can find a willing volunteer, you will probably find the session gets off to a far more positive start.

You can try to persuade the group to volunteer. There are a few things you can say, in order to encourage people to take the seat ... try the following (if they are true, of course!):

'This is not an exercise in ritual humiliation! We are all – you, the simulated patient and me – working together to explore and develop understanding about interpersonal communication. There are no categorically correct answers and we are not here to judge one another. We are simply trying to identify aspects of consultation techniques that are more helpful than others in given situations.'

'This is a group process. The person in the consulting chair is not alone, but is simply working as the mouthpiece for the rest of you, who will be giving suggestions and support throughout.'

'There is no pressure. We just need someone to start us off. You can take time out at any point . . . even if you come up here, introduce yourself and then your mind goes blank, you can take time out. We will stop the consultation, have a discussion together and you can then carry on if you want to, or someone else can take over.'

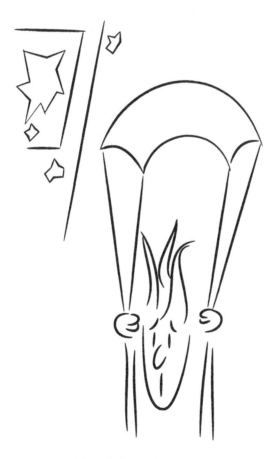

**The willing volunteer!**

'You are not role-playing . . . you are just being yourself, doing just what you would do in your normal day-to-day work . . .'

'Everybody is going to have a turn . . .'

'You have to do this in order to progress to the next year of the course!' [that one always works well!]

'Someone has to do it!' [as desperation begins to set in!]

If your pleas continue to fall on deaf ears, you may offer to start the consultation off yourself, or ask one of the other simulated patients (if there are any!) to play the part of the interviewing practitioner. This can be useful to get the group involved in the scenario, and you can then stop it after a few moments and get someone to swap places with you or the simulated practitioner. They are often more willing by this stage, or else someone in the group feels sufficient pity for your plight that they volunteer in order to save you further embarrassment!

My favourite method, and the one that I find most useful, is to tell the group that I am just going to have a word with the simulated patient outside the room. I ask them to decide who is going to start off the consultation and set the room up while I am doing so. This implies an expectation that they have to find a volunteer from among themselves, and, as you are handing the responsibility over to them, it relieves you from what can be an awkward and even stressful situation. You may return to find they have torched the room and escaped out of the window . . . but, on the whole, it has worked well for me so far!

# CHAPTER 8

# Communication with your simulated patient

*Individually, we are one drop. Together, we are an ocean.*

Ryunosuke Satoro

There are several elements that combine to make for a successful simulated patient session, but one of the most important is (yes, you've guessed it) the simulated patient!

The success of the session can be influenced enormously by the amount of effort you put into communicating with your simulated patient. You are working as a team, and the more you understand about each other's needs, expectations and capabilities, the more effectively you will be able to deliver a robust and enjoyable learning experience.

If you know your simulated patient and have worked with them before, you will already have a relationship to build on, but you should always see it as an ongoing process. There are always points to discuss and clarify with each other, and things to learn from each other. If you are working with someone for the first time, you will need to put in more effort initially, in order to establish the relationship so that you can feel comfortable and confident working with each other.

You should always try to talk with your simulated patient before and after the session, and sometimes it may be necessary to communicate with them during the consultation period. You should be aware, during these conversations, that there is a possibility that the simulated patient may a little overawed in relation to you as the facilitator. This is based both on my memories of my own feelings when I began working as a simulated patient and on many, many comments I have since heard over the years.

Simulated patients may be reluctant to challenge your ideas or requests, and it is important that you try to empower them and give them the confidence to have an honest and real conversation with you. You need to make them feel comfortable enough to refuse any requests that you may have which they do not feel able to fulfil. It will not be beneficial to the session if you persuade the simulated patient to play a role that is in fact beyond their capabilities or that they feel, for whatever reason, they would rather not play.

Sometimes, for example, they may feel reluctant to take an emotional role that is too close to personal experience. This situation should not arise if they have received the scenario in advance, but if you are doing practitioner-directed sessions, or if you ask them to alter a prepared role significantly, they should have the option of avoiding potentially upsetting scenarios. If such roles are a likely requirement to fulfil the learning outcomes, you should make this clear when you are recruiting or booking your simulated patients.

## BEFORE THE SESSION

You should make sure you endeavour to answer any questions the simulator may have and that you are clear about what contribution you would like them to make to the process. The better your initial communication, the easier it will be to work as an effective team.

The following points give an idea of some of the things it could be useful to discuss, although this will obviously depend on how well you know the simulated patient and how much time you have.

You should always try to ask them whether there are any aspects of the role that need clarifying. These aspects could be clinical, psychological or social details. It is important to try to do this even if you only have a very short time to discuss it, as errors in the interpretation of the scenario brief could have damaging effects on the learning outcomes.

You should make sure your simulated patient has no pre-existing medical conditions which may confuse the practitioners.

You may want to discuss what the learning outcomes of the session are, as this can help the simulated patient to work in such a way to help the achievement of these.

It is also important to identify any particular details, within the scenario, that you would like to be brought out by the simulated patient. These may include, for example, specific references to particular information or, indeed, guidance as to how to answer certain questions in the negative if the practitioner begins to go down the wrong path.

You should give an outline of how you plan to manage the session. This includes, for example:

➤ whether you are going to pause the session or play it straight through
➤ whether the simulated patient will be consulting with one practitioner or several
➤ what you would like them to do during pauses, while the group discuss things during the consultation (Would it create more realism if the simulated patient were to leave the room? Would you prefer that they stay in the room and 'freeze', i.e. sit quietly in role neutral? Do you feel it would benefit the discussion if they stayed in the room and joined in?)

➤ how and when you would like them to deliver feedback (there is more detail about the options for giving feedback in chapters 4 and 11)
➤ whether they will be consulting with one practitioner or several
➤ whether you intend to hot-seat them or use any other different techniques.

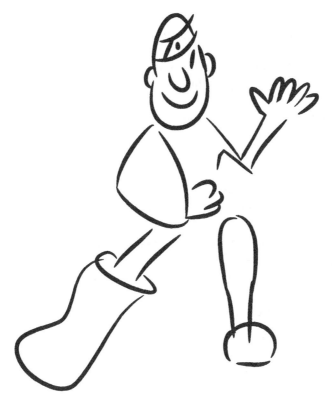

**'I've got this terrible cold, doctor . . .!'**

You should discuss how challenging you would like the consultation to be. This may include aspects such as how readily you would like the simulated patient to divulge information or it may be a matter of what sort of emotions you would like them to express. They should already have an idea of this from the scenario they have had to develop, but it is always worth reiterating, since the level of emotion expressed often dictates the level of challenge presented to the practitioner. A scale of 1–10 can be helpful to indicate the degree of emotion and this can be changed during the session.

You should also try to give a clear idea of how you would like the emotion to be demonstrated. If the scenario is to give the practitioner experience in dealing with aggression, how would you like the aggression to be expressed? For example, do you want quiet, cold anger or loud threats of violence? If it is a bad news scenario, do you want tears or shocked silence? Do you want the simulated patient to walk out of the session at any point or to remain to give the practitioner a chance to sort it out?

It can be helpful to discuss the following with the group:

➤ What professions are they from?

➤ What level of training/experience do the group members have (in descriptive terms, rather than just a number or acronym)?

➤ What are your expectations of a group of practitioners working at that level (although you may be clear what is expected of a general practitioner registrar, not all simulated patients will know!)?

➤ What are the group dynamics like? Is it a lively group or are they a group of treacle waders?

➤ How confident or skilled is the practitioner with whom the simulated patient will be consulting?

## DURING THE SESSION

Once the session has started it is still important to communicate with your simulated patient, although obviously you will have to be more subtle in the way you do this.

There are different reasons you may feel the need to communicate with your simulated patient. For example:

➤ You may want to ask them to vary or adjust the way they are playing the role.

➤ You may want to ask them to increase or decrease the level of challenge for a particular practitioner.

➤ You may be concerned that they are not interpreting the role in a way that is helpful for the group. Perhaps they are leading them down the wrong diagnostic path or perhaps they are taking the focus away from some crucial psychosocial issue.

➤ You may want to discuss the session as a whole. It may be that the scenario is not actually working in terms of the learning outcomes you are hoping for. You may wish to ask the simulated patient to create an entirely new role. This is a possibility for some simulators, but it is important that you negotiate this with them so that they feel confident and are able to portray the role effectively.

There are no easy ways to communicate with the simulator during the session, and the methods you choose will depend on the extent of communication that is needed.

If you have worked with the simulator before, you may find that you can communicate huge amounts simply by body language and the expression on your face, but you will need to be careful that this is not misinterpreted, either by the simulated patient or by the group observing.

You may need to actually speak to the simulated patient at some stage, and how and where you do this will depend on the type of session you are running.

If, for example you are in a practitioner-directed session, there would probably be no problem with simply talking with the simulated patient, in the room, with the group present. In other situations it may be more appropriate to go outside the room with them, briefly. If you choose this option, be sure to explain what you are doing to the group to prevent unnecessary anxieties.

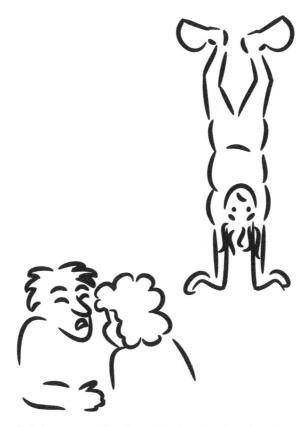

**Subtle communication with the simulated patient**

## AFTER THE SESSION

If it is possible, there is much to be gained from a debrief with the simulated patient after the session. Reflection is always an essential tool for learning and development.

Check whether the simulated patient had any issues about the following points.

### The scenario

You can find out how effective they felt the scenario was. Also, you can find out if there are any significant changes that need to be made to improve the scenario or to make it more effective or easy for a simulated patient to play in the future.

### The organisation of the session

You can find out if there were any aspects of the process that were awkward for the simulated patient, or if they have any ideas for improvements, based on their own experience.

### The group

You can discuss the dynamics of the group, and identify any problems with the participants. This will be especially helpful if it is a group that you are working with on an ongoing basis. It can also be useful after a one-off session as it may help you to identify strategies that may be useful for dealing with difficult situations in future groups. If you have had a challenging experience with the group, the very act of sharing your feelings with a co-worker can help to give each of you the support you need to process it in a positive way.

### The subject matter

This will probably have become evident within the session, but it may be worth checking that the simulated patient has no residual difficulties with the subject matter of the session. They may need some extra help to de-role properly. It can also be worth exploring if there are any other issues that have arisen around the subject matter (e.g. any ethical issues that perhaps were not raised during the session).

### Your facilitation

Finally, it is very useful to get some feedback on your own performance as a facilitator. Simulated patients often have a great deal of experience of different facilitation styles and can be very useful as a resource for your own professional development. However, as I have mentioned, some simulated patients may feel a little intimidated by you, however harmless you may feel you are! If you would honestly like them to give you feedback, be sure to let them know that your request is genuine and make them feel safe enough to do so. It is often more conducive to gaining meaningful feedback, to ask specific, carefully worded questions.

For example, if you ask:

'What did you think of my facilitation?'

you are likely to get a fairly bland, usually positive response.

On the other hand, if you say:

'The group seemed reluctant to give feedback. In your experience, can you think of anything else I could have done to make the feedback process flow more smoothly?'

you will probably get a more useful reply.

# CHAPTER 9

# The consultation

*Words are, of course, the most*
*powerful drug used by mankind.*

Rudyard Kipling (1865–1936)

So you re-enter the room to find a happy volunteer ready to hoist the anchor, an enthusiastic group and the room ready for an observed consultation!

You will need to decide how much you would like the consulting practitioner and the group to know about the patient before they come in, according to the learning objectives of the session. You then need to make sure that they all receive and are clear about the necessary information.

This can be achieved by asking the practitioner who is starting the consultation to read out the instructions they have been given and any medical notes available. There could be a brief discussion about potential issues, as this initial preparation reflects what would normally happen, albeit within the practitioner's head, in the normal pre-consultation process.

You may ask the practitioner if there is anything they would like help with from their colleagues before the simulated patient comes in. For example, if the task is to explain a procedure, the practitioner may wish to clarify the salient points before they begin. Again, this is relevant to the pre-consultation process, as a practitioner would need to make sure they were sure of the facts before explaining a procedure to a patient. It also gives the group the important message that this is a supportive process.

It may be more appropriate for you to simply present the facts to the group. Perhaps you will just outline the situation. For example:

> 'You have been away on holiday and have just returned to work . . . you go to clean one of the rooms, expecting to find Mrs Crabtree lying in bed.'

> 'You have just been asked to cover yet another shift for your colleague who keeps having time off sick when you are told there is a woman in the waiting room who appears to be distressed and is shouting at the receptionist.'

At this point, it may also be useful to look at any aspects of the way they have chosen to arrange the room and ensure that their decision was a conscious one.

> Once, when working as a simulated patient in a recruitment session for general practitioner registrars, I walked in to meet my second candidate. The first had carried out his consultation with us both sat in fairly close proximity across the corner of the large table that was in the room.
>
> This candidate, however, had chosen to move the furniture in order to have sat himself in the middle of the far side of the rather substantial table! I guess he felt safe, but I can't say it was particularly conducive to an open, relaxed consultation!
>
> This would have been a point for discussion had it been a teaching session.

The next stage would depend on how you have chosen to run the session.

## FACILITATING THE STRAIGHTFORWARD SESSION
### What?
You may decide that the most effective way for a consultation to be run is straight through, with no pauses for discussion and with or without feedback given at the end. The feedback may be given in role, out of role or both.

### Why?
You may choose this method of working for a number of reasons:
> ➤ The objective of the group or of the individual practitioner may be to practise carrying out a consultation from start to finish. Maybe they want to study the structure of a consultation or maybe you feel you need to build the confidence of the practitioners in managing the entire consultation.
> ➤ The practitioner may wish to practise their time-management skills. When practitioners have broken down the components of a consultation and practised them, it is important that they can then prioritise, and fit the whole consultation into a specified time frame.
> ➤ The scenario may take place under exam conditions, either as a practice or as the actual exam.
> ➤ It may simply be that a straight-through session, with structured feedback at the end, is your preferred method of working with your group.

### How?
By clearly establishing the process at the beginning of the session and by using a secure feedback structure at the end, this is in many ways the easiest session to facilitate.

When the consultation is to be carried out by one person, without any breaks or change of practitioner, the feedback usually tends to focus more on that person's own interpersonal skills. For this reason, it is useful to ask if there is anything in particular that they would like to receive feedback on, in addition to anything identified by the group earlier. You could then nominate members of the group to concentrate on that area, or just leave it to the whole group to add it to their observational tasks.

Remind the rest of the group of what they should be doing during the consultation. This may simply be writing down their general observations or it could be any feedback tasks they have been given (*see* Chapter 11).

Ensure the practitioner is fully aware of the purpose of the consultation. If the purpose is simply to gather a history, they may stumble if they begin to make differential diagnoses or negotiate a management plan. If the purpose is to negotiate lifestyle changes, then it may be better that they know not to spend a long time taking a full and detailed history.

At the last minute before the simulated patient is invited in, you should always check how the practitioner is feeling, that they think they have enough information and make sure they feel ready to start.

Ask the practitioner to invite the patient in and carry out the consultation, from beginning to end.

Occasionally, practitioners who have worked with simulated patients before in a stop-start session may feel rather daunted at the prospect of managing the whole consultation without being able to pause and discuss their difficulties with their colleagues. In this situation, as long as there was no absolute necessity (such as an assessment) why they couldn't pause for assistance, you could tell them that they may stop if they really needed to. You should try to encourage them to try their best to manage the whole consultation. Often, however, just the knowledge that they can stop if they really need to is enough to boost their confidence to carry out the consultation from start to finish.

You should always write down your own observations in order to be able to structure the feedback at the end of the session. I usually find it most useful to take copious notes, verbatim when possible, highlighting any points that seem relevant to feedback. More information on managing feedback can be found in Chapter 11.

## FACILITATING THE STOP-START SESSION
### What?
Imagine an entire consultation as a video. It may be paused, it may be replayed, it may be fast-forwarded; but, unlike a video, the replays can be varied and different approaches can be tried. This is the stop-start session using a simulated patient.

The potential for learning and practice is enormous but requires great energy, expertise and confidence to make it work well. A stop-start session would most often take place in a small-group setting, with the group sitting in a horseshoe layout around a consulting area to observe proceedings.

The consultation begins and can then be paused at any point for discussion. It can also be replayed in a different way or with a different practitioner, or fast-forwarded to look at a different stage in the procedure. The beauty of it is that the practitioners can try out many different strategies and the group can look at the effectiveness of each one to explore various ways of managing the challenge of the consultation.

## Why?
➤ You may have decided to have a stop-start session in order to allow pauses for discussion.
➤ You may wish to allow for changes of the practitioner carrying out the consultation. This may be in order to give all or many of the group members a chance to carry out part of the consultation, or it may be to encourage a group approach rather than an individual approach to a challenge.
➤ You may wish to introduce variations into the role that the simulated patient is playing. This may be to introduce different learning points, or to alter the intensity of the situation depending on individual practitioner needs.
➤ You can use a stop-start technique in order to allow practitioners to try out different approaches and strategies, or simply to highlight learning points as they emerge.
➤ You can use the method to allow exploration of a more long-term approach to a patient's care, by fast-forwarding to a future consultation.
➤ You can even use it to allow practitioners to explore interpersonal communications that they feel they would never be able to use in reality. For example, they may wish to tell a senior colleague exactly what they think of them. Even though they may never feel able to do this in reality without risking their job, a simulated senior colleague can give them the experience of at least exploring how it might feel were they given this opportunity! This can lead to interesting insights into practitioners' psychological motivators.

The possibilities are endless, but it is perhaps one of the most challenging kinds of session for the facilitator, as well as for the simulated patient. It will require the greatest amount of flexibility and creativity on the part of the facilitator, the simulator and the practitioners themselves in order to be as effective as possible.

## How?
You need to be absolutely sure of certain details of the process you intend to follow. You should not only be clear in your own mind but also make it clear to the simulated patient and the group members exactly how you envisage the session working, before the start of the session. Some of the things that are useful to clarify, as well as a general overview of the process, include:
➤ Who can pause the consultation and how.
➤ The purpose of stopping the consultation.

➤ Whether there can be a change in practitioner when the consultation is paused.
➤ Where the session can be restarted from.
➤ How the consultation is to be resumed.
➤ What will happen with the simulated patient during pauses.

### Who can pause the consultation and how?

You should make it clear that in a stop-start session there is always the option for the practitioner carrying out the consultation to stop the proceedings and ask for time out at any point. This often gives the practitioner more confidence in starting a consultation, if they know they can ask for help if they need it.

They may decide to pause it because they are not sure where to go next with the consultation, and would like to ask their colleagues for some suggestions. They may feel that they would like to try a different strategy.

If the practitioner carrying out the consultation asks for time out, it is a good idea to ask them why they have done so, even if it seems obvious. You may assume, for example, that they are feeling intimidated by an over-assertive simulated patient, but they may feel fine about that and simply be worrying that they forgot to ask for consent for a procedure!

When they have told the group why they wanted to stop the conversation, it is helpful to encourage them to find possible outcomes to their difficulties themselves. It is less detrimental to their confidence if they can come up with their own solutions. You should check out their suggestions with the rest of the group, and gather opinions about the viability of their ideas. It may also be useful at this stage to see if anyone else in the group has any other thoughts or suggestions.

Your own ideas, however brilliant, should be put on a back burner, only to be used in case of emergency! As a facilitator, it is easy to get so involved in the session that you wish to enthusiastically impart your own pearls of wisdom and suggest strategies or make comments, especially if the group is a little lacklustre. Take a deep breath and ask the group for their ideas first. You can prompt and guide them, but the more of the 'work' they can do for themselves, the deeper, richer and more robust their learning will be.

If it is a session where more than one group member can be involved in each consultation, you may offer the consulting practitioner the choice at this stage of carrying on themselves or of swapping with someone else. It can be helpful, especially if there has been a fair amount of discussion, for you to summarise the options that have been suggested. You can then ask the practitioner who is going to continue the consultation to choose one or more of the strategies identified by the group that they feel that they would like to try. This gives them an opportunity to clarify the next stage in their mind before resuming the interaction.

If there have been many useful strategies suggested, perhaps the practitioner, or different group members, may like to try out different potential solutions to the same problem. This can work very well, though you must make it clear to the simulated patient that they are going to be repeating the same part of the consultation a number of times, in order to explore the different outcomes. In this case you would return to the same moment in the consultation to try each suggestion.

You should make it clear that you, as the facilitator, may stop the session to highlight learning points or facilitate discussion. You should explain that if you do stop the consultation, it is not necessarily a reflection on how well the practitioner is doing, but that you simply feel it is a useful place to pause for discussion. You may decide to stop it for a number of reasons:

➤ There may be a specific learning point that you have identified that you feel would be useful to highlight and discuss with the group.

➤ You may feel that the practitioner is finding it challenging and rather than letting them struggle on, some suggestions from their colleagues may help them move it forwards.

➤ You may feel that the consultation, for whatever reason, has become diverted from a helpful course. This could be because some unexpected emotional response from the simulated patient has affected the interviewing practitioner. It could be that the practitioner has misinterpreted some clinical information and is going down the wrong path.

➤ You may wish to ask the simulated patient to alter the way they are playing the role, to make it more or less challenging.

➤ You may simply want more members of the group to have a go at consulting with the patient. If you do decide that it would be beneficial to the process for someone else to continue the consultation, you must suggest this sensitively. It is important that the practitioner who is standing down should not feel as though they have 'done it wrong' and that is why someone else is taking over.

➤ You may be aware of time constraints and wish to move the consultation on to a later point, or even to fast-forward it to a follow-up consultation in the future.

➤ You will have already decided on the input you would like from the simulated patient during the session. It can occasionally be useful during discussion to ask for their comments on specific points of debate that may arise. I would recommend, should you choose to do this, that you keep them in role and keep it brief, just to inform your discussion with the simulated patient's perspective.

➤ You may decide that it would be helpful to extend the right of pausing the consultation to the other members of the group. This may be for different reasons:
  — they may have an idea about where the practitioner could take the consultation
  — they may have some strategy for dealing with a particular difficulty
  — they may simply wish to try a slightly different approach.

You should be very clear that this is how you would like to run the session, as it can make proceedings quite difficult to manage if all group members are able to stop the consultation at any point. You should be very clear at the beginning of the session about the purpose and procedure of this. How would they go about this? Should they indicate to you that they have a suggestion to make, or can they simply stop the proceedings by announcing 'time out'? You should be clear about the purpose of this, while emphasising once more that everyone needs to be mindful of the principles of good feedback at all times.

I would recommend that you do not allow the simulated patient to stop the consultation at any point. It is usually preferable that the simulated patient stays in role at all times, unless you ask them to come out of role.

The only time it may possibly be necessary for the simulator to ask for time out is if you are doing a practitioner-directed session and they need some additional information. This should have been negotiated and agreed with the group at the beginning of the session and should, in any case, be avoided if at all possible.

There are exceptions to this, as in all aspects of simulated patient work, which we will look at later, but as a general rule it is better to keep the simulator in role until directed otherwise.

## Simulated patient in pause mode

You will need to decide what you want the simulated patient to do when the session is stopped.

You have several options. First, you can ask the simulator to leave the room while the discussion between the practitioners is taking place. They should leave the room still in role, wait until called back in, and then return still in role.

Another option is to ask them to stay in the room, in role and 'freeze' in role neutral.

It should have been explained to them in training that they are not 'freezing' in a dramatic way but they should relax a little and be still, perhaps lowering their gaze to the floor to avoid making eye contact with anyone in the group.

> I remember during one particular workshop about defusing violence and aggression, the situation had escalated considerably. I was virtually nose to nose with the practitioner, threatening him with all kinds of unpleasant retribution . . . when suddenly the facilitator paused the scenario. I froze. She wanted to discuss the situation with the group, leaving me and the unfortunate general practitioner gazing into each other's eyes, at very close proximity, for what seemed like an eternity! (I think it was probably only a couple of minutes!) What should have been a passing moment of aggression and intimidation acquired some uncomfortably intimate overtones and thoughts of garlic and raw onions! This is why I would now recommend relaxing and averting your gaze during a pause; you never know how long they are going to last!

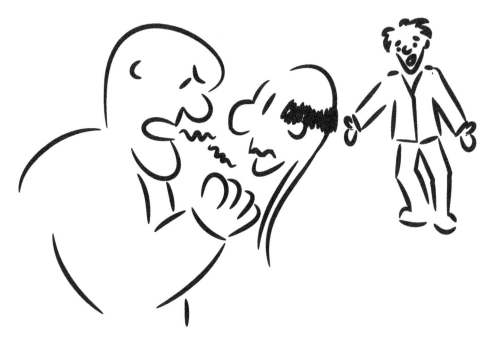

**OK, let's pause it there . . .!**

Another option is to ask them to stay in the room and join in the discussion. This can be in role, whereby you, the practitioner carrying out the consultation or a member of the group can ask their character questions about how they feel about certain aspects of the consultation. This can be very helpful, and practitioners can check out their assumptions as the consultation progresses. You should encourage the simulated patient to limit their comments at this point to the specific questions that are being discussed. It can also be out of role, whereby you invite the simulated patient to come out of role in order to join in with the discussion. I would not recommend this, as it may then be more difficult for the simulator to resume the consultation. It usually adds confusion to the situation, and as a general rule out-of-role feedback and discussion should be kept until the end of the consultation.

There are advantages and disadvantages to either keeping the simulator in the room or asking them to leave during a pause. If they stay in the room, they will hear the discussion that takes place, giving them an idea of the group's ideas and expectations, as well as the state of mind of the practitioner carrying out the consultation. It may be appropriate for them to adapt their reactions according to what they have heard . . . or it may be inappropriate. Ask them simply to be aware that they may be doing it, in order to make it a constructive, conscious decision! You should also explain to the group that if the patient is freezing in role neutral that they should behave as though the patient has gone. You must make it clear to them that they can freely discuss any aspects of the consultation, as the simulated patient is, to all intents and purposes, not present.

Alternatively, if the simulator leaves the room, they obviously have no idea about what the group have discussed. It can be argued that this gives a more honest, objective response to the consultation. The practitioners may also feel less inhibited in their discussions if the simulated patient is not present. Even though they know that the simulator is not the real patient, they still sometimes feel awkward discussing their character while they are physically in the room.

Leaving the room takes longer, so if you have many pauses for discussion, this can take considerable time from your session.

You may decide a combination is appropriate. For example, if the practitioner pauses proceedings simply to ask a brief question, perhaps the simulated patient can sit in the room, but then if the whole group need to discuss management options, perhaps it would be less appropriate for the simulator to hear those discussions.

You need to consider the advantages and disadvantages of each and decide which would be most useful for the particular session you are running. Whichever method or combination of methods you decide to use, it is important that you make clear to both the simulated patient and the group exactly what will happen.

### Restarting the consultation

If the simulated patient has gone out of the room during the pause, after discussing consultation options within the group you may need to go out of the room to speak to them to give them an idea of what you would like them to do as the consultation resumes. You may wish to indicate the content of some of the discussions. You will need to tell them if there are any changes in the way they are playing the role, whether you would like there to be a greater or lesser challenge, or if the character is to be played in a different way or in a different situation. You will also need to tell them where they will continue the consultation from. You can then return to the room and ask the practitioner to call the patient back in.

If you do not speak with the simulated patient during the pause and simply send the practitioner to call them back in when you are ready, the simulated patient will assume that there are no changes to be made and that they will be resuming the consultation from the point it was left off.

If the simulated patient has been in the room during the pause, they will obviously be aware of the discussion and the plan of the group. You can simply invite them to restart the consultation, and they should look up again and begin the consultation from the point indicated.

You may wish to ask the simulated patient to repeat the last line to restart the consultation, or the practitioner may start proceedings. You may choose a part in the consultation where things started to become difficult and ask the simulated patient to repeat a line from there.

If there has been a change of practitioner in the meantime, you need to decide how best to deal with this. Do you want them to introduce themselves to the patient, or should they carry on as though they are the same practitioner? This again should be made clear to the group and to the simulated patient.

A useful way to restart proceedings, especially if there has been a change of consulting personnel, is to get the practitioner to give a brief summary of what has been discussed so far in the consultation.

### Replaying the consultation

As we have seen, we can replay a consultation with a simulated patient much as we can replay a video. The difference is that a video can only be replayed in the way it was recorded, whereas a consultation with a simulated patient may evolve in many different ways when it is replayed.

You may ask the simulated patient to go right back to the beginning of the consultation or you may ask them to begin at a specific point. You may ask them to play it in a different way – for example, slightly more anxiously, or less talkatively.

Make sure they realise that this is not necessarily a criticism of the way they have been playing it; it is simply to give the group a different experience. Perhaps a practitioner needs a slightly more challenging situation. Perhaps the practitioners have swapped during the pause and you feel that the needs of the new consulting practitioner are different. Perhaps you have a specific teaching point you would like to illustrate.

### Fast-forwarding the consultation

Sometimes you may find it useful to move to a later point within the consultation. This may be for various reasons. For example, if the group's objectives are to practise ending a consultation, there is little point in spending a lot of time on introductions and history taking.

Alternatively, the consultation may have been challenging and provoked a great deal of debate and discussion. You may feel that you would like the practitioners to tackle another aspect of the consultation and so decide to move it forward to the management planning stage.

Sometimes it may even be useful to move to a subsequent consultation. In this case you should ask your simulated patient to take a moment to imagine how their character is feeling a week later, for example. As the moods, expectations and so forth of patients change between consultations, then so must those of their character. You must remember to give the simulated patient some guidance as to what may have happened in the intervening period and how they may be feeling now. For example:

> 'You have taken all the medication as prescribed and nothing seems to have made any difference, so now you are feeling really fed up and want something done about it.'

> 'In the meantime, you have found out that it was heart disease that killed your aunt, and so now you are angry that the doctor doesn't seem to be taking you seriously.'

This enables the simulated patient to know how they are supposed to react in this follow-up appointment.

You should also ensure that the consulting practitioner knows what they would realistically be aware of, in the intervening period. For example, they may have no idea what has happened to the patient in the intervening period, or they may be aware that they have attended outpatients or had some diagnostic tests performed. They may or may not have the results of these, but they should be aware of this.

As mentioned earlier, this kind of session can be challenging for the simulated patient. Some suggestions for ways in which you can ask them to vary their role, increasing or decreasing the complexity, may be found in Chapter 4.

## SIMULATING RELATIVES AND THIRD-PARTY SESSIONS

The term 'simulated patient' is, to a large extent, a misnomer. Simulated patients can play the part of patients, relatives or health professionals (although there are potential training implications to this last one – *see* Chapter 4). If you require a simulator to take the part of a patient's relative, you can point out to them that the difference is really only in the content of the scenario. There is no difference in the actual manner of working to playing a simulated patient in different situations, when they are working alone in a session. Instead of responding to questions about their own health, they will be discussing the welfare of a relative.

This can be used to explore many communication issues. It may be that the group want to practise different ways of dealing with an angry person, in which case perhaps they can be asked to complain about the treatment a relative has received. It may be that the practitioners wish to look at some ethical considerations, so they may be asked to discuss something about a relative that is perhaps confidential, or they may be asked to give consent for a procedure on a relative.

You may decide it is useful for the simulated patient to play a relative or friend when the 'patient' is in the consultation too (or they may play the patient 'wedded to' or the 'spawn of' another simulated patient!).

This allows the practitioners to practise consulting with two people at the same time. This may be a parent and child (although, currently, because of difficulties in working with children, the 'child' would normally, but not always, be played by someone over the age of 16), other relatives, a heterosexual or homosexual couple, or friends. The extra difficulties presented when consulting with more than one person are often exaggerated in these scenarios. This could be by having one person dominating the other, or for some reason perhaps the person who is playing the patient has some physical or psychological difficulty in communicating.

It is important when creating a third-party session to allow time for the two simulated patients to establish their relationship with each other! They need to know about factual issues (e.g. if they are a married couple, do they have any children? What ages are the children? Do they both work?). They also need to understand certain psychological issues (e.g. if one is the patient, how does their partner feel about their illness? How is the relationship between them? Do they have any secrets from each other? Are there additional stresses affecting either of them?). They should have time to practise how to behave together, how to relate to each other. They should have a few brief conversations with each other in role, to get used to how each reacts to different things.

It is important when working with a partner that they can trust each other, in order to make the situation realistic.

Once the scenario begins, it should progress as normal, but the main difference then comes in feedback, when you will need to ask both parties to comment. As well as the usual issues simulators may be asked to give feedback on, a three-way consultation involves some extra challenges that require comment. These may include, for example, what strategies the practitioner used and how successful they were in managing to involve both parties in the consultation, seating arrangements, eye contact and so forth. Third-party sessions can be quite challenging but are very rewarding and good fun when you are working with two simulators who can realistically portray the subtleties of a relationship.

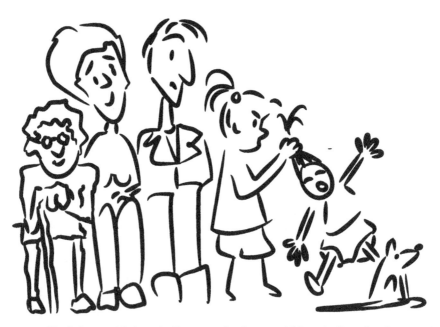

**'And they said the triadic consultation could be challenging!'**

## BILINGUAL SESSIONS

One increasingly common use of third-party scenarios is where an interpreter is needed to enable the practitioner to consult with the patient. This may be when a patient does not speak English fluently.

For this work you will need to recruit simulated patients who speak English and another language fluently. The second language is necessary for the playing of the scenario, but it is essential that they speak fluent English as well to enable them to give sensitive and constructive feedback.

These scenarios may take different forms. There is scope, obviously, for different characters to be used and different challenges to be presented, but the emphasis is usually on the actual problems of communicating with someone via an interpreter.

There are a number of situations you may wish to present to the practitioners. The most straightforward scenario is where a practitioner employs the services of a professional interpreter. You may ask one simulated patient to take the part of the patient who speaks no English, and the other to play the part of the interpreter. Ideally, the simulated patient should be trained to portray professional interpreting standards. This means that they must interpret the exact words that are said, and this should be done impartially, completely and objectively. When anything is said by the practitioner or by the patient, the interpreter should interpret it using the first person, rather than reporting it in the third person. For example, instead of reporting:

> 'The nurse wants to know what's wrong.'

or

> 'She says she's got a really bad pain in her stomach.'

they should translate directly:

> 'Hello, Mrs Orlicka. What has brought you here today?'

or

> 'I have a tummy ache, it's really bad.'

The practitioners may be practising using a professional telephone interpreting service. You can therefore ask one of the simulated patients to take the part of a patient who has to communicate with the practitioner by passing a telephone backwards and forwards, and speaking to an unseen complete stranger. The other may play the part of the professional interpreter, again translating accurately, impartially, completely and objectively. This type of session presents practical difficulties regarding use of equipment, and you will need to make decisions about how best to manage the situation. Further discussion on this subject can be found in the section on facilitating telephone consultations later in this chapter. This consultation, using a telephone interpreting service, should raise some of the same difficulties of a standard telephone consultation, but some slightly different issues should also be highlighted. The practitioner should at least be able to communicate non-verbally with the patient, although the use of the equipment and the fact that all verbal communication is via an unseen stranger will present plenty of other challenges.

The practitioners may be exploring the potential difficulties experienced when a patient who speaks no English brings a relative along to interpret for them. In this case, the scenarios themselves or the way you ask the simulated patients to portray the characters can provide a variety of learning points for discussion. For example, you may ask one simulator to portray a relative with a fixed view of the problem or a patient vulnerable in the hands of an overbearing relative. You may choose to ask the simulator playing the relative to report the conversation in a selective manner, including their own issues in this and making their own judgements about what is being said. If this is the case, guidance should be given in their brief about it, but you should also describe exactly what learning points you are hoping to illustrate, before the session begins. For example, if the patient says,

> 'I haven't been able to go to the toilet for a week now.'

the simulator playing the family member may choose to interpret it as:

> 'She's got problems down below . . . it's all the junk food she eats.'

If they are 'misinterpreting', adding or leaving out information, they should try to make this quite clear in the consultation. For example:

Practitioner:   'So how long have these problems been going on?'
Relative:   (to patient) 'She wants to know how long you've been getting them for . . .'
Patient:   (to relative) 'Well, I've been getting the headaches for ages now. I was already getting them before I left Bahrain, so that must be at least 6 months now . . . I just didn't have a chance to get to see a doctor out there because we were getting ready to move . . . it was all very difficult . . .'
Relative:   (to patient) 'So, why didn't you come as soon as you arrived here then if you'd already been getting them for that long?'
Patient:   (to relative) 'Well, then, I wasn't sure if I'd have to pay to see a doctor over here, and you know I don't have the money for that, so I didn't come for ages . . . but they've got so bad now, I've just had to come because I'm so worried . . .'
Relative:   (to practitioner) 'Six months.'

The practitioners may be looking at some of the issues arising when no professional interpreter is available and they have to use a member of staff, with greater or lesser command of the language spoken by the patient. You can, once more, encourage the simulator playing the interpreter in this situation to use tactics to emphasise learning points as above, and also make it clear that there are things that they are not quite sure how to translate.

There may also be ethical issues, for example around confidentiality, which you can ask the simulator playing the interpreter to emphasise in the way they portray the character. Again, this should be indicated in the scenario, as well as verbally before the session begins.

The practitioners may want to attempt to communicate with someone with very limited English, but without using anyone to interpret for them. You may then ask the simulated patient to pretend to be a patient who has very poor command of English but is trying to manage to communicate alone.

Apart from the normal consultation skills issues arising from non-bilingual sessions, these difficult situations raise many different issues – practical, psychological, social and ethical! These range from confidentiality to the difficulty in making an accurate diagnosis when the practitioner cannot be certain that they have complete or true information; from the balance of power within relationships to how best to arrange the seating to engage with the patient; from culturally acceptable practices to deciding where the practitioner should direct their eye contact during the consultation.

One of the specific challenges in performing bilingual simulated patient work (apart from finding effective simulators who are also able to speak two languages fluently!) comes in giving in-role feedback. Further information on the simulated

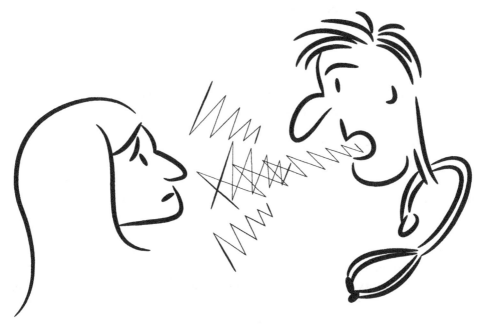

'Where exactly can you feel the pain?'
'I thinking . . . three weeks doctor . . .'

patient giving feedback can be found in Chapter 4. Feedback clearly needs to be given in English, but it can be very challenging for the simulated patient to remain in role and yet suddenly speak a different language. Some people feel comfortable remaining in role and switching to fluent English. Others prefer to imagine they have just had 6 months' intensive language classes and their command of English has improved dramatically, but they are still clearly from the designated country. It may sometimes simply work better to ask the simulated patient to come out of role for feedback. You should always make it very clear to the simulator which of these you would like them to do. You should also endeavour to listen to the simulated patient's personal preference during your discussions, as it can be such a tricky area for them to manage.

As more health professionals are recruited from overseas, there is an increasing need for specialised sessions to meet their particular training needs. These sessions are similar to standard teaching sessions, the main differences being, much as they are in bilingual scenarios, that feedback tends to be focused on quite specific communication areas and there may be cultural considerations to explore. For example, often discussion focuses on forms of greeting or use of non-verbal communication. There is often exploration of how much explanation a health practitioner should give about their own communication difficulties. For example:

> 'Good morning, My name is Magda Szypczynska and I have recently come to work here from Poland. I know that my English is not perfect and please . . . if I do not understand everything you say . . . be patient with me. If you do not understand what I am saying, please ask me. I'm sure together we will manage!'

In this way, the health professional is inviting the patient to be understanding of the difficulties right from the beginning, which often eases the situation and should lead to a more open consultation with a clearer outcome.

### SIMULATING HEALTH PROFESSIONALS
Although the majority of the work that simulated patients are asked to do involves portraying a patient in consultation with a health professional, you may find it very useful to create a situation in which the practitioner can explore ways to deal with challenges arising within their relationship with another health professional.

This could be used in training workshops for professional appraisal, interviewing techniques or perhaps conflict management. You may even ask a small group of simulators to play the part of professionals taking part in a meeting of some kind, to look at problems with team-working, management issues or perhaps the perspective of the service user.

Although the principles of working as a simulated patient and the mechanisms for feedback are essentially the same when portraying a health professional as when portraying a patient or relative, you should be aware that this situation does present particular challenges for the simulated patient.

We all (unless we have been very fortunate indeed!) have some experience of being a patient. We do not all have experience of working as a particular health professional. Each profession has its own jargon and its own procedures. Each professional has his or her own training and experience.

A simulated health professional needs to present a convincing portrayal of a social worker, nurse, doctor and so forth without this knowledge or background. Not only that, they will probably be working with a group of people belonging to that profession, or with experience of working with that profession, who do know the jargon and procedures and who do have the training and experience. This can make for quite a difficult situation!

It is important that you acknowledge this additional challenge.

➤ When offering the work in advance, emphasise that they can refuse the work, without it jeopardising any future opportunities. As I have mentioned, it is important that they feel comfortable about the roles they accept.

➤ Help them to research their subject. Give them opportunities to talk to professionals, or talk to them yourself about the role you are asking them to portray. Guide them towards websites, written or artistic material that may give them insights into the role.

➤ Encourage them to ask any questions relating to the situation before the session. Make sure they feel as confident as possible about what is expected of them.

➤ Discuss a possible time-out option with them before the session. This would mean that if they were asked a technical question to which they did not know the answer, they could indicate in some way that they needed that information and you could then pause the session to provide the additional guidance.

With experience, simulated patients usually find it becomes easier to simulate health professionals, as they work with them and learn more about their roles and responsibilities, and the language they use.

If simulated patients are involved in practitioner-directed scenarios, they may be asked to take the part of a health professional. In this case, you will probably have involved them in the devising of the scenario in some way and they should have had the opportunity to ask their questions there. It may be useful to highlight the difficulties to the group yourself and to ask the practitioners themselves to suggest actual words or phrases to help. It is important in this situation to devise a time-out facility for the simulated patient, should they need more information during the course of the interaction.

## CAMEOS

In some ways this is the simplest way for a simulated patient to work. It can perhaps best be described as a mini-performance.

Most simulated patient work is extremely interactive and the learning takes place within the interaction. The cameo, however, is far less so, and is used mainly to demonstrate a point rather than to explore it. Cameos may be used during a conference to focus the delegates' minds on the issues being discussed, they may be used to illustrate points raised by a speaker giving a presentation, or they may be used as an energy-raiser after lunch at a conference.

A cameo is usually short and is often prepared to some degree. This could be in the form of a mini-play with a number of performers, a dialogue or a monologue. It could be scripted, semi-scripted or improvised. The cameo may simply be presented with yourself or another member of the facilitation team, with another simulated patient or with a previously chosen 'briefed' member of the audience as the practitioner.

Ideally you should give the simulated patient access to the presentation notes beforehand to give them a clear picture of some of the issues that you are planning to highlight. You should also give clear guidelines as to your expectations at each part of the presentation; for example, will you want comment in role or out of role at any point? How should they behave if the presentation is paused?

You can also use cameos on the rare occasion when the participants of a teaching session feel unable to take part in a consultation. You can ask the simulated patients to perform the consultation with one simulated patient (or, indeed, yourself) playing the part of the consulting practitioner, and the other playing the part of the patient.

While this may be necessary on occasion, it should only be used as a last resort, as more effective learning takes place through interaction than observation. If you do need to resort to this under such circumstances, it is usually more helpful if there are some clearly ineffective behaviours demonstrated by the person playing the practitioner. Always take an early time out for discussion, and, having become involved in exploring different strategies, one of the group members may at this point feel happier to become more actively involved and the session can progress as normal.

## TELEPHONE CONSULTATIONS

As has already been noted, the use of simulated patients is limited by imagination alone, and it is important to keep a close eye on developments within healthcare practice, in order to provide training according to needs. An example of this is the rise in the use of telephone consultations.

Training in consulting with a patient, relative or colleague over the phone can be useful in a variety of settings; for example, for receptionists dealing with an angry patient, for general practitioners assessing a depressed patient, for junior doctors who are requesting the attendance of a reluctant on-call consultant or, as we have seen, for practitioners using a telephone interpreting service.

Basically, the principles of working with a simulated patient in a telephone consultation are the same, but they will be unable to see the consulting practitioner, and the practitioner will have no sight of the simulated patient.

The way you arrange this will depend on the resources you have available, and on the learning outcomes of the group. You may have a telephone link to another room with a loudspeaker facility. In this way the group will only see the body language of one of the participants but will hear the entire consultation. The practitioner is usually the person who stays in the room with the rest of the group, but it may be useful for the patient to be the one the group observes. It may even be possible to split the group physically and have half watching the practitioner and half watching the patient.

You may have a telephone link to another room, but with no loudspeaker facility. In this case, the group can watch one person's body language but can only hear half the conversation. Again, this would usually be the practitioner, but it may be interesting to watch the patient. In a bilingual session, the group would be able to observe different body languages and non-verbal communication between the practitioner and the patient, and it would be interesting, if possible, to observe the difference it makes using the handset with or without loudspeaker facility.

You may have no access to telephones, in which case the practitioner and patient would need to be divided by a screen or sit back to back. This situation has benefits although, it loses realism in that the group can then watch and listen to the whole interaction and observe strategies and the reactions to those strategies.

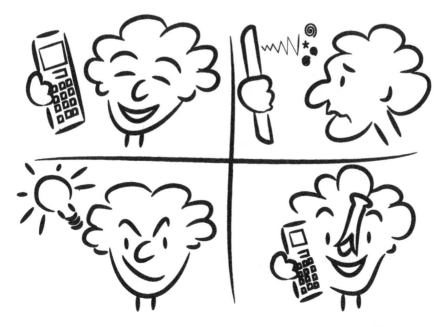

**'The number you have dialled has not been recognised.'**

It is interesting to note the challenges this kind of situation provides. With no body language, including facial expression, to help them, the practitioner still has to assess the situation and mood of the character. The simulated patient also has no body language on which to assess the consultation, so they must make a careful analysis of the language and tone of voice that the practitioner uses, in order to give constructive feedback.

A useful exercise is to arrange for some of the group to turn around so they are facing away and then observe aurally. This can add another dimension to feedback.

## CO-WORKING WITH HIGH-FIDELITY MANNEQUINS

Darling! They told you never to work with children or animals . . . but did they ever mention big plastic dummies with pulses, blinking eyes and a tendency to go into cardiac failure at the drop of a hat?

Resusci Anne, the mannequin used in first aid training courses for years, has come a long way from her somewhat humble origins! Modern mannequins are produced in a large variety of shapes and sizes, from bodybuilders to babies, disembodied ears or armpits to the odd pet dog! They are now able to reproduce many bodily functions, such as breathing, blinking and bleeding, and they can respond in real time to medical intervention. They can also be linked to monitors, which can provide a realistic situation for teams of health professionals to deal with in training. They are used much more extensively these days to train people to deal with medical emergencies of different kinds. Although the focus of this book is on working with human simulators rather than high-fidelity mannequins, you may find yourself presented with the opportunity of working with such a resource.

The most frequent use of combined human and low-fidelity mannequin simulators is in assessment situations when the candidates are required to undertake an intimate examination or when they are supposed to find an abnormality. Simulated patients and high-fidelity mannequins are more frequently used in teaching scenarios.

Many medical emergencies are accompanied by distressed relatives, and so you may wish to ask a simulated patient to play the part of the relative or friend, giving the practitioners the chance to practise dealing with the medical situation while attending to the emotions it arouses in others.

This is an exciting new development that offers huge potential for integrating clinical skills and sophisticated communication skills in a realistic combination.

## PRACTITIONER-DIRECTED SESSIONS

These are also known as masterclasses, improvised sessions or practitioner-led sessions.

There is a definite movement towards practitioner-directed sessions. They are a great way of ensuring that you are addressing the specific needs of the group.

If you have the opportunity, and feel you have the confidence, I would urge you to consider offering the chance for at least one of the consultations within your session/s to be generated from actual difficulties encountered, or even just witnessed, by members of your group.

It is useful to give the practitioners in your group advanced notice of this option. This enables them to actively look out for situations they may encounter in practice that could provide useful learning material. These may be situations the practitioners themselves have experienced, or they may be incidents they have simply witnessed. Often communication difficulties occur not with patients, but with relatives and also with other professionals. It is very useful to be able to explore these situations in practitioner-directed sessions, and you should remind the group of this option as they are initially thinking of potential scenarios. You could do this either by telling them in an earlier session, or even by sending a letter or email before the session if you are unable to speak with them. Such contact before a session also acts as an initial warm-up as practitioners begin to think of communication difficulties and focus on the issues.

If you don't have the opportunity to give advance warning (or even if you do!) it is helpful to allow a few minutes at the beginning of the session for the practitioners to speak with each other, in pairs or small groups, about actual or potentially challenging situations they have encountered in practice. They can then bring their discussions to the larger group. The simulated patient can sometimes be involved in these sessions, right from the outset, or they can be brought in after this initial discussion with the group.

Whichever of these options you choose, you can then write each situation on a flip chart, discussing and noting the main difficulties within each. You could try at this point to identify issues and themes that are common to more than one person's experience. This is an important stage, as it is essential that you and your group identify the underlying communication issues, rather than becoming focused on the actual circumstances of the original interactions themselves. The identified issues then become the communication challenges of this group, some of which can be explored during the session. Learning objectives can be developed from these suggestions.

You should then identify who will carry out the consultation. This could be the person who was involved in the original interaction or it could be someone else. There are pros and cons to each and you should decide which would be best according to the situation. For example, the practitioner who was involved in the original situation may not be able to move away from the actual events surrounding that incident in general, or they may even still be traumatised by the situation. However, the danger of inviting another practitioner to carry out the consultation is that this could make the original practitioner feel they had 'got it wrong'. Once more, it is important that you, as the facilitator, emphasise that this is simply an exploration of the difficulties and that there are no right or wrong answers. You could offer the originating practitioner the chance to start the consultation, but then, just as in a normal stop-start session, you can swap the consulting practitioners to allow different people to try different strategies.

At this point it is useful for the volunteer to leave the room and wait outside and the simulated patient to be invited in if they weren't already in the room as a part of the original discussions. The rest of the group are then given the task to devise a useful scenario, with the simulated patient, to present to their colleague. This is often where the frustrated authors and film directors come into their own! While a lot of fun can be had concocting challenging plot lines and characters, it is important to make sure they do not forget some of the basic essential facts! You may decide to write these on a flip chart, to make sure they have all been covered. It is important, also, that the group do not get too carried away with high drama to the detriment of the learning outcomes sought.

Consider which of the following basic facts would be useful to include:
➤ which parties are involved and why they are having this interaction
➤ the main problem
➤ background to the main problem.

If it is a consultation with a patient:
➤ main health issue
➤ any other health issues
➤ past medical history and family history
➤ medications and allergies
➤ their social circumstances
➤ their main ideas, concerns and expectations
➤ their basic frame of mind and how they are likely to behave during the consultation.

If it is a consultation with a relative:
➤ main health issues of patient
➤ the relationship between them
➤ their feelings for each other
➤ their social circumstances
➤ their main ideas, concerns and expectations
➤ their basic frame of mind and how they are likely to behave during the consultation.

If it is to be an encounter with a colleague:
➤ their main duties
➤ their relationship to the practitioner carrying out the consultation
➤ any issues they may have with them based on the original story
➤ any relevant jargon
➤ any personal background that could contribute to the problems
➤ any other information that would help the scenario run smoothly.

Always make sure that you give the simulated patient the opportunity to ask as many questions as they wish, so that they can feel confident in portraying the role. Experienced simulators can virtually facilitate the role-development part themselves, but you must make sure that they do get enough information and that they and the group remain focused on the desired learning outcomes. When you are sure that the simulated patient is happy with the role and the situation, you should ask them to wait outside and invite the poor unsuspecting practitioner to come back in.

The group will outline the basic situation: where the interaction takes place, any relevant history, any particular factors that the practitioner would be aware of. They should only give information that the practitioner would realistically know if it were a real situation.

The practitioner would then invite the simulated patient in as usual and begin the consultation.

The session would continue in the usual way, but you should bear in mind that if you decide to allow another member of the group to take over the consulting for any part of the consultation, they will already have additional background information.

You should also remember when planning these sessions that they require the simulated patient to have excellent improvisation skills. There is a very short time in which the simulator can develop and learn all aspects of their character, so they need to be able to work quickly and creatively. Always encourage them to ask as many questions as they need to in order to develop a convincing and useful role.

It is essential that you make sure that the simulated patient is happy and confident with the scenario and can give a convincing portrayal. This is especially challenging when they are asked to play a colleague. They are then expected to assimilate a degree of understanding of the role of the professional, as well as the jargon that person may use and the characteristics they may have. For this reason, this is one of the rare occasions when you can allow the simulated patient, if absolutely necessary, to take time out, during the consultation if they do not understand something. You may also decide that a certain amount of 'direction' is appropriate, to be given by the rest of the group, both before the consultation, and if necessary during it.

In my experience, groups are always able, with the right encouragement, to identify suitable challenges from practice. If you are feeling insecure with the idea of practitioners creating their own scenarios, I would recommend giving it a go, but having some ideas of your own that you can have ready to suggest to get the ball rolling. If you are feeling really panicky, you could actually have a scenario already prepared with the simulated patient, to be used as a last resort. However, I would encourage you to do your best to facilitate the generation of practitioners' own scenarios.

At the end of the session, it is useful to check that the scenario developed did in fact fulfil the learning objectives identified during the original discussions.

Sometimes it is possible to address more than one issue within each consultation. For example, if one practitioner had highlighted a difficulty with dealing with an angry patient and another had struggled with being put in a position where their professional integrity was brought into question, it should be possible for the scenario to include a patient or relative who wished to complain about the behaviour of another member of staff.

It can be helpful at the end of the session, as well as revisiting the learning outcomes to ensure they have been met, to revisit each specific communication challenge. The strategies tried by the practitioners can then be identified, and the more successful ones can be recorded as tangible outcomes for the session.

Practitioner-directed sessions often evaluate very well as they can be pertinent, challenging and fun!

> Some time ago, I was working as a simulated patient with some fourth-year medical students. A situation that one of the students had found difficult while on clinical placement was an interview with an elderly, slightly deaf, very confused patient, who seemed unable to understand what he was asking her. Initially I tried to play the patient as he had described her but, whether due to my lack of acting ability or simply to my comparatively youthful (hmmm!) appearance, it seemed to be difficult not to parody the situation. The old lady became too much of a caricature to enable effective learning. I then tried to identify the main issues the student had found difficult – communication difficulties and slightly bizarre behaviour – and created a different character (a woman under the influence of drugs) that was more believable and which still illustrated the main challenges. This time, the consultation was more effective in allowing the student to explore different ways of dealing with this situation. This illustrates the importance of trying to get to the core of the actual communication issue, rather than trying to recreate the details of a specific challenging consultation.

## REMEDIAL SESSIONS

Occasionally, an individual healthcare professional may be identified as having particular difficulties with one or more aspects of their consultation or interpersonal skills. If it is felt that they would benefit from some extra help, it can be quite useful to arrange a simulated patient session, which could be focused on their specific requirements.

This could be for a number of reasons. They may be a student who has failed an examination because of poor communication skills. They may be a practitioner from overseas who needs some extra help to carry out a consultation in the way in which it is expected to be carried out in this country. They may be a practitioner who has received complaints against them and, as part of a remedial process, it is felt that they need some extra training in consultation skills.

(A far higher percentage of doctors who are forbidden to practise medicine lose their registration because of communication difficulties than because of clinical incompetence.) They may have some physical impairment which makes communication more of a challenge for them.

You should initially spend some time in discussion with the practitioner in order to assess what the particular difficulties are and, crucially, how much insight they have into those difficulties. You then have a choice. You could either write some scenarios that you feel would provide the practitioner with the opportunity to explore those difficulties and improve their skills or, alternatively, and probably preferably, you can invite them to attend an individual improvised session with a simulated patient.

Here, you would discuss the issues with the practitioner and the simulated patient, and together would devise some scenarios that would potentially address some of the difficulties. This is an unusual situation to be working in as there would be no group to give feedback, and so it is important to be able to sensitively challenge the student to evaluate their own performance, as well as feeling confident to give strong positive and constructive feedback yourself.

It is also essential that you find a very experienced simulated patient whom you can trust to give sensitive feedback that will build up the confidence and skills of the practitioner.

## HOT-SEATING

As we have seen in Chapter 4, hot-seating is often used by simulated patients as a way of building up a character; however, as a technique it also has many applications within teaching sessions. It is a useful method of speeding up the process of gathering information about the patient's character and situation.

It can be used effectively for a number of reasons and it can be used at different points within the session. I will outline the process and explore some of the reasons hot-seating can be useful.

First, you should explain to the group the purpose of using this method. It is useful, for example, if the scenario involves a patient who is supposed to be known to the practitioner and they would therefore need some information in order to assume this relationship. Although mock medical notes can give some information, it would not necessarily give the practitioner a picture of the person's life or personality that can be more effectively gained through hot-seating.

You may choose to do it in order, for example, to gather a medical history quickly, to enable the group to move on to the management planning part of the consultation. For example, if the focus of the session is on negotiating treatment options with the patient, it is important that not too much time is spent on gathering a history to allow enough time for the negotiation stage. If practitioners need to practise ending a consultation, there is little point in spending a great deal of time on taking a detailed history. However, if you do decide to hot-seat for this reason, you should ensure that the practitioner still has the opportunity to build a rapport with the patient before launching into tricky negotiations, for example.

Hot-seating can also be used before or during the feedback session, in order to discover any salient points that did not come out in the course of the interview. You would need to do this sensitively, with regard to the feelings of the practitioner/s who had carried out the consultation. They should not feel they have failed if certain information has not come to light. The simulated patient may have had instructions in their brief not to divulge particular pieces of information. They would, however, be able to talk about them in hot-seating, as they would be in role neutral (more about this presently). It can be a useful discussion point for the group to identify challenges within the consultation and to think of how, if ever, certain information can be elicited.

Hot-seating could also be useful in enabling an exploration of different ways of asking questions, which may result in the patient revealing other pieces of information more readily, or identifying some underlying issues that perhaps there wasn't time to discover during the course of the consultation.

Sometimes there are pieces of information or underlying issues that do not seem to be emerging during the course of the consultation and which are essential for the group to know in order to meet their learning outcomes. You may decide in this instance to pause the consultation and let the group hot-seat the patient in the middle of the session. The practitioner/s can then continue with the additional information to finish the consultation.

You may decide, if you are short of time, to interrupt the consultation and use hot-seating simply as a method to speed up the information-gathering process.

Hot-seating is often used, as we shall see, as an integral part of forum theatre in order for the practitioners to gain more insight into the life situation, personalities and motivations of the characters involved.

You should also explain that the simulated patient is in role neutral. This basically means that although they are still in role, they are without the extremes of emotion that may become evident in the scenario or may have been experienced in the scenario (depending on when you choose to introduce the hot-seating). So if the character is reluctant to disclose information in the scenario, they will be more open in hot-seating. If they are angry in the scenario, they will be calmer in hot-seating.

Once you have ensured that the group are clear about the reasons you have chosen to use this method, you should ask the practitioners to fire questions at the character to find out any information they would like to know. These questions can be about anything, including their social situation, their medical history, their emotional state and so forth. They may be asked to describe a particular experience or their feelings about a particular incident. The questions can be about anything, but will tend to focus on the group's task in hand.

Encourage the practitioners to simply call out their questions rather than taking turns. This, again, keeps the process rapid and energised and encourages all group members to ask the questions they would like to know the answers to. Use eye contact and phrases such as:

'Anything else?'

or

'Come on, more questions . . .'

to encourage all participants to join in.

You can chip in with your own questions when appropriate, in order to model the kinds of questions you would like them to ask, to ensure that essential information is discovered and to keep the process lively.

You should encourage the practitioners to ask the questions fairly randomly. Although this goes against the grain of what we normally teach about structure, it is important to keep the information moving quite quickly. There can be a tendency, through familiarity, for practitioners to drift into taking a medical history. This can be one practitioner getting carried away, or the group taking it sequentially. You can ask other questions to divert this process, or simply remind them that they are not supposed to be taking a structured history.

It is better to encourage each person to ask a maximum of two or three questions at a time. This also discourages the practitioners from falling into the trap of taking a history, or simply of asking too many questions on one particular topic. Hot-seating is an incredibly useful technique, but should be used intelligently and sparingly to avoid the risk of the session losing structure and focus on its objectives.

## FACILITATING LARGE GROUPS: FORUM THEATRE

If you have a larger group to work with, it is worth thinking of different ways of managing the session. A standard personal interaction may be more difficult to facilitate in a large group, for many reasons. Logistically, it is more difficult to find suitable accommodation that would enable the practitioners in the group to be both in audience mode and in interactive mode. Also, a practitioner who may have no qualms about volunteering in a group of eight to ten trusted colleagues may be less keen to show off their skills in front of an audience of 250!

There are many different possibilities, limited again only by the imagination (and possible environmental considerations!).

You may decide to facilitate a forum-style session. This is a less intimidating way of involving a group with a communications process. As practitioners are critically observing problematic behaviours, they can often recognise difficulties in communication without actually having to own the difficulties for themselves. This makes it an effective way of exploring problems without causing practitioners to feel vulnerable or exposed in any way.

Forum theatre was developed in the 1950s and 1960s by the Brazilian theatre director Augusto Boal. Initially known as Theatre of the Oppressed, it was created as a way of giving a voice to those who struggled to be heard. His initial directives are interpreted in a variety of different ways these days, and forum

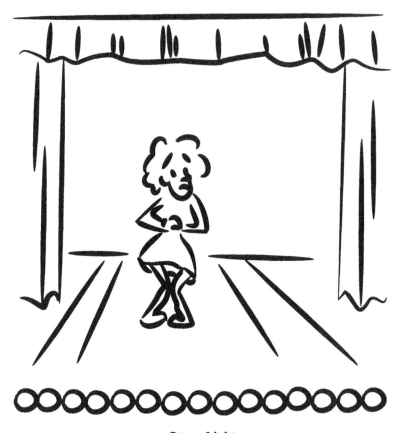

**Stage fright**

theatre is widely used as a training method. I will describe one method I have been involved with extensively; however, I would like to stress that you may be asked to vary aspects of this procedure, according to the style of the facilitator or the needs of the group.

Ask the simulated patients to act out a scenario, either fully scripted or improvised, but with clear communication issues.

Stop the scenario after a few minutes. After a brief discussion about the main issues, divide the practitioners into groups, according to the number of characters in the scenario. Three is a usual number, but there are no hard and fast rules about this. Each group will then be allocated one simulated patient.

The simulated patients would normally remain in role throughout, but it may occasionally be deemed preferable for them to speak with the group out of role. The following description assumes the simulated patients are still in role.

What happens next may vary slightly, but will usually begin with some hot-seating, where each group's members ask their simulated patient some questions to try to find out a little more about their character and their character's life. They will be trying to discover something of the character's motivations for behaving in the way in which they behaved in the scenario. The group may also want to find out about any background issues that may account for the character's atti-tude within the scenario. For this reason, even if the scenario is fully scripted, it is very important that the simulated patients are also confident about their knowledge of the details of their character's life and personality.

Each simulated patient will then ask their group for some guidance on how to proceed to get the best out of the situation. The group members can give the simulated patient advice, but they cannot change the basic personality of that character. You may need to guide them gently to help them to understand the difference.

With the directions each character has received, they then return to the sce-nario and continue to act it out from the point at which it was stopped.

You can then explain that the scenario may be stopped again, but that this time it is up to the practitioners to stop the action if they feel their character is not carrying out their directions, or if the behaviour of one of the other char-acters is preventing their character from carrying out the directions they have been given.

Each simulated patient will then return either to the same group or, more usefully, you can send them to a different group to receive further advice and direction. Each group has the best interests of the character whom they are cur-rently 'directing' at heart.

This process may be repeated several times.

There may be discussion afterwards or at various points during the session about some of the issues raised. You may at this point be asked to give feedback, either in or out of role.

If you choose to facilitate a forum theatre session it is helpful to remember a number of points. For example, point out that no one will be expected to parti-cipate in the actual scenario itself (unless they desperately want to!); rather, they will assume the roles of directors. This usually relaxes the group and they are able to engage with the process almost immediately.

You should also emphasise the fact that the situation will not be resolved. It is more about exploring some of the issues that underpin difficult interactions, and gaining some insight into various perspectives on communication challenges. Some useful approaches will be identified, but it is unlikely that there will be time to reach resolution, if one were ever possible.

You need to be aware of the impact of the action on the group throughout a forum session, as it is within this that much of the learning takes place. You may choose to give the 'audience' tasks, such as Edward de Bono's Six Hats Exercise (*see* Appendix 6) while they are watching the initial performance, but usually the issues presented are quite clear and often quite dramatic enough that this is not necessary.

During subsequent performances, each group tends to be focused very much on what their 'character' is doing and how the others are treating them. They are concerned as to whether they are following the group's directions and, if so, with what success. One of the important tasks of the facilitator of a forum session is to make it very clear to the participants what they should be doing when they are in their small groups with their actor. First, they should hot-seat the character, in order to learn more about the motivations behind their behaviour. You should then instruct the groups to give their character advice on how to proceed within the interaction from the point at which it was stopped. You need to emphasise that the personality of the character cannot change, as in reality people do not change their personalities dramatically in an instant. The character may be able to change their behaviour, but only within the bounds of their fundamental personality.

You need to gauge how long to leave the actors with their groups, depending on how complex the issues involved are, how much time you have for the session and how well the groups are responding to the task. Before the action is resumed, you should hand over responsibility for stopping the action to the audience. From this point in proceedings, they are in charge. They are allowed to stop the performance:
➤ if they feel their character is not carrying out their directions
➤ if they feel their character is being compromised by the other characters
➤ if they feel the situation is getting out of control again for whatever reason.

You may need to be ready to stop the action yourself, but in my experience this has never happened, as the participants usually become very involved in the process. Forum theatre is a very engaging, fun way for practitioners to work with simulated patients, and by this stage they have usually become very much a part of the 'action' without the need for further encouragement.

You can repeat the process, moving the actors from group to group, as many times as seems appropriate. Sometimes it is appropriate to let all participants see the situation from every character's point of view; sometimes it is enough just to swap once or twice.

Forum theatre is often useful as a warm-up activity in order to prepare a group for more interactive and in-depth work. Sometimes it is the main way of working for an entire session. The practitioners may become more involved, depending on how the session develops.

I recently attended a session for young people with diabetes that involved a scripted piece wherein a girl with diabetes attends a routine clinic with her mother. The scene demonstrated some of the difficulties inherent in the situation, and the problems that arise within the relationships among the people involved, despite the best efforts of those involved. The young people in the group were able to identify with the frustrations of the girl, but were also able to gain some insight into the challenges facing the parent and the consultant. When the scripted part ended and the forum discussion began, the young people were very enthusiastic to take over the parts of the simulated patients and the improvised part of the scenario ended up being acted out by the young people themselves!

Sometimes the term 'forum theatre' is used to describe any form of interactive training using actors or simulated patients. This may include anything from a straightforward goldfish-bowl style of working, whereby the scene is presented and then questions and directions are taken from the group, to a situation where the group develop a scene to illustrate their own learning outcome needs.

You could provide the simulated patients with a character scenario, as well as a sequential storyline, with a number of scenes. These could be written as outlines of the situation presented. Each scene would potentially present a variety of communication and ethical challenges. The group would then be divided according to the number of scenes involved, and they would be asked to examine the issues raised and devise some strategies that could effectively be employed by the practitioner. A volunteer from each group would then perform the role of the practitioner with the simulated patients in roles of patients, relatives or colleagues. The success of the strategies could then be analysed by the whole group.

As ever, the possibilities are endless. The main thing you should do before running a forum session is to make an honest appraisal of your own skills, experience and confidence as a facilitator. Working intimately with a small group of practitioners, focusing on individual micro-skills, is a very different situation to organising a large group into subgroups and facilitating discussions and interactions on such a big scale. However, it is a challenging, fun and very interesting way to work with a larger group of people or with a less confident group.

## FACILITATING MULTIPLE GROUPS
If you are in the position of being responsible for more than one group (oh yes, it happens!), there are a number of options.

➤ You could try to identify any group member/s who possibly have more experience of working with simulated patients and ask them if they could take the role of facilitator within that group.
➤ You could ask one or more of the groups to facilitate themselves (if they are experienced in this way of working), while you facilitate another group.
➤ You could ask more than one group to facilitate themselves and you could 'float' in and out of each group, to ensure continuity and to emphasise relevant learning points.
➤ You could ask the simulated patient if they would feel confident to facilitate the sessions themselves. This is extremely difficult if you are hoping for a stop-start session. If you have to use this option, it is easier simply to have the consultation carried out from start to finish and then ask the simulated patient to lead the feedback session. However, as we shall see in Chapter 10, self-facilitation is extremely challenging and it should only be the most experienced simulated patients who are asked to do it.

Whichever of these options you decide to choose, it is even more important than normal to emphasise points of process before the beginning of the session. The practitioners should be very clear about the learning aims of the session, the process of the consultation and the structure of feedback. This should help enable the groups to take more responsibility for their own learning, as they will be more confident about the task and how to approach it.

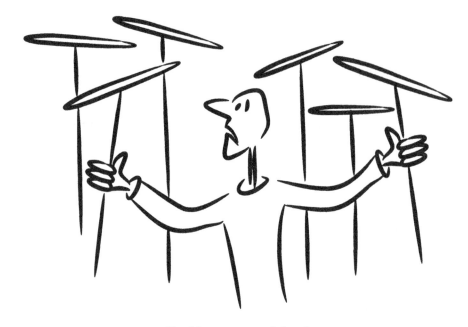

**'And for my next trick . . .'**

## SIMULATING PHYSICAL SIGNS AND SYMPTOMS

While simulated patients are commonly used to assist in the development or assessment of a practitioner's consultation and interpersonal skills, they can also be very useful in teaching and assessing diagnostic and examination skills.

You have many options for the teaching of clinical skills, and a combination of a variety of different methods is obviously the ideal. However, the option of using simulated patients is still underutilised for a variety of reasons and the potential is still largely to be explored.

A simulated patient can be trained to understand the anatomy and pathology linked with a certain condition and can then reproduce the signs that would indicate a problem. For example, if you wanted to teach practitioners to diagnose problems with the hip joint, you could train the simulated patient to adopt the relevant gait, and demonstrate the precise amounts of flexion, abduction, rotation and so forth, as well as give an accurate indication of when and where the pain occurs. In this way, the practitioners can gain experience in actually physically examining a patient, as well as integrating their diagnostic skills with interpersonal communication, which they will have to do in reality.

Such examinations can and should obviously also be carried out on real patients with the condition. However, the advantages of using simulated patients on occasion include the following:

> ➤ a real patient who is experiencing pain may suffer in the hands of an insensitive practitioner
> ➤ a real patient may not be able to withstand examination by large numbers of practitioners
> ➤ a real patient may not be able to give the practitioner focused feedback
> ➤ a real patient may not be able to understand the integrated nature of examination skills and give feedback appropriately.

Some physical symptoms (e.g. pain and stiffness) are quite easy to simulate. Others (e.g. bruising or rashes) can be demonstrated with a little bit of preparation. There are also simple techniques that can be used to simulate other physical signs and symptoms; for example, clenching one's buttocks can apparently increase blood pressure!

You may also involve simulated patients in more elaborate simulation events, whereby, with the use of make-up and prosthetics, they present a person with a specific type of illness or someone who has had, for example, a road traffic accident. They may then be 'attached' to monitoring and life maintenance equipment. The readings on this machinery could be adjusted to create a variety of situations that the practitioners would need to deal with. This allows health professionals to practise their assessment, monitoring and emergency care skills in a realistic setting, integrating clinical competence with communication skills with a real person.

Such simulations are also useful in helping practitioners to look at different aspects of team-working and inter-professional communication. Teams of practitioners can develop their skills and understanding together.

### THE USE OF VIDEO WITHIN SIMULATED PATIENT SESSIONS

The use of video (and, to a lesser extent, audio recordings) within consultation skills training sessions involving simulated patients is an invaluable resource for the practitioners. It can be used in many different ways, although the way you may choose to use it may depend largely on the technological resources available to you.

The video may be used within the session to record all or part of a consultation. It can then be replayed within the session, at a later session or by the practitioner in their own time. It can provide valuable visual evidence of the practitioner's skills and areas for development. In sessions where you replay and review the video, you can invite simulated patients to comment on communication skills demonstrated. If any difficulties are identified, you can also ask them to improvise a situation to allow the practitioner to explore other ways of dealing with the challenges they experienced in the original interaction. The feedback may also be recorded to provide additional learning material at a later date.

Recording the session provides the opportunity for clear self-observation and reflection. It also provides the possibility of reinforcing the learning from the session by using a more formal reflective assessment in which the practitioners can analyse their consultation and discuss the feedback received.

The use of video creates a record for the practitioners of their consultation, and this can be reviewed and examined many times. It gives them a level by which they can monitor their own progress.

Observations made by the simulated patient, the facilitator or the other group members can be reinforced if the practitioner is later able to watch a recording of their consultation and identify, with the benefit of hindsight and the feedback received, those behaviours that brought about a positive response and those that perhaps were less helpful.

The session may be recorded to allow the practitioner, as part of an ongoing process, to reflect on their work and their progress in a more formalised way. This may be a written reflection, to enable trainers to assess the learning that is taking place within the group and by each individual.

A video of the consultation can also assist in the giving of descriptive feedback, either during the session or at a later date. Accurate references can be made to specific points, phrases or behaviours within the consultation. This is easier than relying on your own or the group's collective memory, which therefore makes the analysis of the skills and behaviours used more accurate.

It allows flexibility in your organisation of the teaching session. You can (technology allowing) have the interviewing practitioner in one room carrying out the consultation with the simulated patient. You can be in another room with the group of observers, watching the interaction. This adds greater realism to the simulated situation, as the practitioner is not distracted by a group of colleagues watching, and it allows you to highlight behaviours with the observing group as they occur.

You may decide to make training videos using simulated patients. These can be used in future consultation teaching sessions to illustrate certain learning points. It can be cheaper to use pre-recorded videos rather than using simulated patients every time, although (as I hope you will have realised by now) this would offer a very different experience to the practitioners. If you decide to make a training video using simulated patients, you may like to involve them in the process of designing the video (with regard to props, clothing and so forth).

Training videos can also be used to train assessors for examinations, to help achieve consistency in their approach to marking.

You may decide to record some or all of the stations in an examination. This can be used to ensure consistency in the simulated patients' performance and to make sure that the marking is fair and appropriate to the situation.

You may need to check out the rules as regards filming a simulated patient. As a general rule, as long as the video is purely used for in-house educational purposes, there should be no problem. If it is to be used in a more public arena, you will probably have to pay them standard filming rates. Emphasise to the simulated patients, however, that they are still effectively a learning tool for health professionals – they don't need to worry about presenting their 'best side', for example . . . in this instance they are unlikely to be 'spotted' by any Hollywood scouts!

So we have seen that video is an invaluable aid to consultation skills training. For a practitioner to actually be able to observe their own performance, especially after they have received comprehensive feedback on their skills, is a very powerful tool. However, I must stress that video should be used wisely in teaching sessions! You must be aware that you run the risk of losing some of the advantages of working with 'live' simulated patients.

Recording the consultation and then discussing it afterwards moves the learning to the theoretical level to some extent, since we are then guessing how things could be different. With a stop-start process, the learning is very much kept in the experiential, as difficulties can be identified and explored as they occur, rather than through analysis after the event.

If you have the facilities available and decide to use the video in another room from the group, you can bring the patient back through in role afterwards, to allow an exploration of challenging parts and in-role feedback.

Where simulated patients can be used in the analysis of a recorded session, whether immediately after the session or at a later date at a review session, this allows opportunities to explore and practise some of the issues raised by the recording.

A combination of the 'live' simulated patient session with a simple recording of the whole process can be very useful.

# CHAPTER 10

# The simulated patient as teacher

As with any resource, it is worth exploring the potential in order to maximise the benefits. Simulated patients can be expected to take a greater or lesser role within any teaching session, and they can also receive additional training in order to allow them to assume more responsibility within teaching or assessment.

## CO-FACILITATION

All consultation skills sessions involving a simulated patient and a facilitator should be a partnership. The two people involved have different roles within the session and will ideally work closely together to deliver the most effective learning experience for the practitioners.

In practice, the interpretation of this partnership can vary enormously. Sometimes you may simply expect the simulator to perform a role in a cameo, as an illustration of a point you wish to make or to promote discussion. In other teaching sessions you may want them to act as a co-teacher and expect them to have a far greater and more proactive role in managing feedback and entering discussion.

In discussion with the simulated patient before every session, you should clarify the level of involvement you are expecting and ideally evaluate it afterwards. Ultimately you, as the facilitator, are the person who understands the aims and objectives of the session, and even the dynamics and individual strengths and weaknesses within the group. Therefore, it is important that you are very clear before the session as to your expectations as far as the contribution of the simulated patient goes, beyond the playing of the role.

## SELF-FACILITATION

Occasionally and increasingly, you may need to ask simulated patients to work without a facilitator. This is an extremely challenging situation and one that I would not recommend for inexperienced simulated patients. You are already identifying the complexities of working as a facilitator in a simulated patient teaching session. You are also endeavouring to understand the complexities of working as a simulated patient. Now imagine doing both jobs at the same time! It requires the simulators to be able to work on an even greater number of different levels simultaneously than they do when working in a normal simulated patient situation. It is as though they need to hide a teacher's hat inside whichever character they may be playing!

The simulated patient, as we have seen, has a very complex role within the teaching scenario. If you can imagine, while fulfilling the demands of this role, also being aware of, for example, the dynamics of the group, the aims and objectives of the teaching session, the needs of individual group members as well as the group as a whole, the process and their own contribution to that process, both as simulated patient and facilitator, well, that will give you some idea of the challenge that self-facilitation presents!

There is an increasing amount of institutions currently experimenting with different models of working without a facilitator. These include studies that give groups of practitioners the task of running their own session without a facilitator. This happens after the process has been carefully modelled and strategies developed to assist them in managing their own learning.

Other models include pilots of sessions where the simulated patient manages the session as well as acting as the patient. A simulated patient may be asked to manage a one-to-one or one-to-two session, within which they would facilitate learning outcomes as well as take the part of the patient. This can be a very effective way of learning, but it relies entirely on the expertise of the simulated patient and the maturity of the learners.

Although some institutions do value this as an effective model to use, sometimes the decision to use this model is in response to economic constraints, as the full simulated patient process is relatively expensive to use. It can also be developed in recognition of the trend towards practitioner-directed learning. It is a difficult process for the simulated patient, and compromises often have to be made. If you ask a simulator to be involved in this kind of session, please consider the following:

➤ Make sure they are not afraid to say no! Some simulated patients will be more at ease with this role than others because of past experience and other acquired skills. As with all aspects of simulated patient work, it is essential that they feel competent and confident with the situation before they accept the work.

➤ If they do decide to accept the challenge, ensure that you clearly explain the teaching aims of the session and that they feel comfortable with the process. They are effectively the teacher.

➤ Remind them to use clear signals as to their status (as simulated patient in role, as simulated patient out of role or as facilitator).

➤ Encourage them to spend plenty of time explaining the process carefully and thoroughly at the beginning. They should ensure that the group understands not only the aims and objectives of the session but also the potential ways the session could be run.

➤ Ask them to try to encourage the group to take responsibility for the running of the session and for their own learning within it. It is often worth them asking for a volunteer from the group, perhaps one who has previous experience of working with simulated patients, to take the responsibilities of facilitator while the simulated patient is in role. This relieves them of the anxiety of working out when to pause the session, and generally overseeing proceedings, at least while they are involved in the consultation.

## ASSOCIATE CLINICAL EDUCATORS

Also known as clinical teaching associates or clinical teaching assistants, these are simulated patients who have received extra training in order for them to become competent in assessing or teaching basic physical examination skills. They can learn how a correct examination should be carried out and how it should feel to a patient. They are then able to teach practitioners the best ways of carrying out the examination, giving accurate feedback on aspects of their clinical competence as well as their interpersonal communication skills and how it feels for the patient physically.

Gynaecological teaching assistants are simulated patients who have received additional training to enable them to teach practitioners to carry out intimate examinations, including pelvic examinations. Working in pairs, they allow the practitioners to perform the internal examinations and are then able to give feedback on both the practical aspects of the experience as well as the interpersonal skills they have demonstrated.

As it is such a valuable experience for learners to actually gain feedback on their practical skills, their communication skills and the integration of the two, this is an area that is expanding. Obviously, it is crucial that you recruit simulated patients with the skills and experience to enable them to perform these tasks competently:

➤ They must feel comfortable with the experience.
➤ They must receive adequate training in the relevant medical details before embarking on such work.
➤ They must be clear about how the ideal examination should be conducted. This is in terms of procedure as well as technique.
➤ They must be sensitive to the practitioners' potential embarrassment as examinations, especially intimate examinations, are carried out for the first time. They must, as should everyone working in potentially sensitive areas, be wary of becoming blasé about the experience. It will always be the first time for some practitioners and the difficulty should always be acknowledged.
➤ They must have teaching skills, as they need to convey information to students about the procedure as well as give feedback about their interpersonal skills.

# CHAPTER 11

# Managing feedback

*For there is nothing either good or*
*bad, but thinking makes it so.*

William Shakespeare (1564–1616)

The most essential part of the session is the giving of feedback. This is where most of the learning takes place and is reinforced. This is where the practitioners gain insight into their behaviours, their strengths and their areas for improvement.

There are many different theories around the most effective ways of giving feedback; however, common to all is the principle that it should be a positive and constructive experience, both for the person receiving the feedback and for those giving it. There are many models for ways of managing the feedback part of the session. A variety of factors will influence which particular model or amalgamation of models you consider to be the most useful.

As facilitator, it is your job to ensure that the experience of receiving feedback is a positive one for each practitioner and you must be certain that every member of the group is aware of his or her responsibility within this. You must make sure they understand the point of giving feedback and are able to do so in a supportive way, which helps their colleagues to learn and grow in their skills and confidence.

One useful analogy I have used is that of the giving of a gift. They should be thinking of what the person would most like to hear and what would be most useful for them, and then they should be presenting it in such a way that would be most pleasing to them. You may also make explicit the point that a gift may be received graciously and appreciated or it can be rejected as it is, in effect, somebody else's idea of what a person may need or like. Ultimately, feedback is an offering and a person cannot be made to respond to it, although they should be encouraged to reflect on it.

During the feedback process, you must remain sensitive to dynamics within the group; should a practitioner receive feedback that is in any way potentially harmful, it is up to you to right the situation, sensitively and respectfully. This can be a delicate situation, but it is crucial that it is well managed for the sake of the individual group members and for the whole process.

While acknowledging that there are many different feedback models, I will reiterate one point that I feel is essential to remember, whichever model or models you choose to use:

> 'The practitioner who has carried out the consultation should always be asked how **they feel** about the consultation, first.'

This is vital to give everyone in the room a clear indication of how the practitioner views their own performance, to enable them to pitch their feedback appropriately. After this, and only after this, should other group members and the simulated patient be asked for their opinions!

## FEEDBACK MODELS

One of the tools to safeguard practitioners is the feedback model. There are numerous such models, each with its own advantages and drawbacks. By rigidly following a model, you are less likely to inadvertently allow a practitioner to fall foul of destructive feedback; however, as in many aspects of life, complete inflexibility can also lead to problems. I would again recommend that you familiarise yourself with a variety of models and techniques to provide yourself with a large toolkit you can use according to the needs of any given situation.

I am going to outline my own interpretation and developments of three of the models most commonly used in a variety of consultation skills training sessions. I describe them in the ways in which I have found them most effective to use. If you would like to understand more about them in their purest form within a theoretical framework, references are given in suggested further reading (*see* Appendix 7).

### A feedback structure based on Pendleton's rules

David Pendleton and colleagues developed Pendleton's rules in 1984, in order to counterbalance the excessively negative feedback that was often given to medical students at the time. Through its structure, it ensures that there is a balance between positive and constructive feedback, as well as trying to ensure safety for the practitioner receiving the feedback. By being given positive comments first, it helps avoid the situation where a practitioner is so demoralised by negative comments that they cannot hear the positive ones, or where they become excessively defensive, making it more difficult to help them see the constructive nature that should be inherent in the process.

As soon as the consultation finishes, ask the practitioner how they are feeling.

You should allow time for this, and even if they are only able to cite the parts that were difficult, allow them full expression of these.

If there were negative points brought out by the practitioner, do not dwell on them at this point. Simply acknowledge them, possibly summarise them to make sure you have understood exactly what they meant and promise that you will return to them presently.

You may feel a temptation to counter their self-criticism at this point, but this is not necessarily helpful. Occasionally, if the practitioner raises a small, straightforward point that you are absolutely sure is simply a case of them being hypercritical, you could quickly ask the group and the simulated patient for brief, specific feedback. For example:

> *Practitioner:* 'I kept on forgetting what I was going to say, it must have looked as though I hadn't a clue what I was doing!'
> *Facilitator:* 'Did the rest of you notice that?'
> *Group member:* 'I did notice you pause a couple of times, but I don't think it looked like you didn't know what you were doing . . .'
> *Facilitator:* 'Can we just check that out with you, Mrs Macintyre? Did Emily seem to know what she was doing?'
> *Simulated patient:* 'Oh yes . . . even when you did pause sometimes, you then went on to ask really sensible-sounding questions . . . I prefer it when a doctor thinks about what they're going to say!'

On the whole, though, it is better simply to acknowledge their worries at this point. Make sure you have noted the points down so that they can be returned to.

Ask the practitioner what they have done that they feel has been helpful in the consultation. At this point, you have a choice. You can ask them for a full list, again acknowledging and noting each comment as it is made, and then return to the list for a fuller discussion with the group when the practitioner has run out of things to say. Alternatively, you can discuss each point with the group as it is made. You can make this judgement each time, depending on the group you are working with and the comments made, and it is not necessary to stick to a hard and fast rule about this.

If you do discuss each point with the group as it is made, I think it can lead to a more inclusive and lively process. It involves the rest of the group in the process immediately and by getting a lively discussion going at this point, the entire session will function at a deeper level as well as at a more enjoyable one.

Invite the rest of the group to identify what they felt went well in the consultation. When the practitioner has raised all the points they were pleased with, you can invite the rest of the group to give their examples of effective practice, with examples, and checking their observations with the simulated patient in role, if you choose to have them do this. For example:

> *Group member:* 'I thought you built a really good rapport with the patient.'
> *Facilitator:* '. . . and what did Ahmed do to build that rapport?'
> *Group member:* '. . . well, he was really friendly when he brought her into the

room . . . and I thought the patient seemed really pleased when he asked her
what sort of dog she had . . . I think that helped to build good rapport . . .'

*Facilitator*  '. . . so, shall we check that out with Mrs Murphy?'

*Group member:*  'Mrs Murphy, it seemed to me that you felt quite relaxed
when you were talking to Ahmed . . . is that right?'

*Simulated patient:*  '(*to practitioner*) Oh yes, I thought you were so friendly,
everything you did really . . . you were smiling, you seemed really interested in me . . . and when you asked about Henry . . . (that's my dog) . . . I
just thought, now here's a chap who can really understand the things that
matter in life!'

Ask the simulated patient, in role, what they felt had gone well. The simulated
patient should be asked if they have anything to add (in role) about what they
felt had been successful, which hasn't already been mentioned. If they have been
verifying the observations of the group throughout the feedback session, they
may have little to add, as they may have expanded on these points as they went
along.

Then you, as facilitator, could share any further thoughts about things you
have noticed that went well in the consultation. Ideally you should have little to
add at this point because you will have helped the practitioners to identify many
of the points already.

You should then ask the practitioner if they felt there was anything they would
like to do differently, if they had a chance to do it again. You could remind the
practitioner of any points they may have brought up at the beginning when you
asked them how they were feeling, and then see if there were any other points
they felt they were not too happy with. With each point they identify, if you ask
them if they have any alternative strategies they feel may have been more effective, it gives them the chance to remedy the situation themselves. If appropriate,
you could rehearse any of their ideas as they are made, with the simulated patient,
to allow the practitioner to experience any differences.

You can ask the rest of the group what they feel about any of the points that
the practitioner identifies. Usually, they are quite kind to their colleagues and
this can be a gentle way to open the discussion and begin an exploration of
alternative approaches. Again, any alternative suggestions can be rehearsed and
explored with the help of the simulated patient. You can, if time allows, invite the
group members to try out any suggestions they have with the simulated patient
themselves, rather than the original practitioner doing it.

Ask the rest of the group if they had noted anything that could be tried
differently.

When all the practitioner's points have been explored, you should ask the
rest of the group if there was anything they felt could have worked better with
a different approach. Again, try to get as specific and descriptive points of feedback as possible, and assumptions can be checked with the simulated patient
throughout.

Ask the simulated patient for any additional comments about what could be tried differently. The simulated patient is invited to give their perspective on things that were less effectively dealt with.

Add any further comments as facilitator. As before, this will be limited, as most of the points should have been covered following your earlier prompting of the practitioners to identify these.

Bring the simulated patient out of role. When everyone has had their chance to give their feedback and explore alternative strategies, you should bring the simulated patient out of role and ask if they have anything else they would like to add about the practitioner or the process.

### A feedback structure based on agenda-led, outcome-based analysis

Some drawbacks to Pendleton's structure were identified, such as its rigidity (although this is often down to interpretation) and the moral weighting placed on the behaviours. Also, by insisting that the positive feedback is heard first we run the risk of a practitioner not being able to concentrate on the positive comments, because they are anxiously anticipating the more constructive comments still to come. In 1996, Jonathan Silverman and colleagues introduced a new model of feedback called 'agenda-led, outcome-based analysis'. This is intended to take the best of Pendleton's rules while minimising the drawbacks. It makes a subtle shift from a judgemental assessment to a more task-based approach.

Before the consultation begins, you should ask the practitioner who is about to carry out the consultation to identify some of their perceived problems. In this way, the group can be looking out for those specific aspects of the consultation as it proceeds. For example:

*Facilitator:* 'Are there any particular aspects of your consultations that you would like specific feedback on?'

*Practitioner:* 'Well, I always struggle to keep to my structure when the patient takes me off down a different path . . . I get engrossed in what they are telling me and forget to ask important biomedical stuff!'

You can then ask the whole group, or particular members of the group, to look out for specific occasions when this occurs and what strategies, if any, the practitioner uses to bring the consultation back on track. If you are able to learn the practitioner's agenda before the session, you can also ask the simulated patient to provide an opportunity for the practitioner to experience this within the consultation. This should be done subtly, but it provides another opportunity to fine-tune the session to meet the learning needs of individual practitioners.

Start with the practitioner's agenda. Immediately after the consultation ends, you should ask the practitioner:

'How do you feel about the consultation?'

'What problems did you encounter?'

'What help would you like to receive from the rest of the group?'

In this way, the feedback will be focused on the practitioner's own perceived needs. It will get straight to the nub of the problem as identified by the practitioner and so will allow them to focus on the feedback. By getting the practitioner to actually specify what kind of help they would like the group to give them, they are less likely to become defensive and will be more able to receive the suggestions.

Identify the outcomes that the practitioner and the patient were hoping to achieve in the consultation. When thinking about strategies to deal with challenges within a consultation, it is always useful to clarify exactly what the practitioner and the patient were trying to achieve. You can explore what the original aims were, and if anything happened during the consultation to alter these. For example, the original aim might have been to explain a procedure to a patient, but the patient is in a state of high anxiety at the thought of the procedure. The main aim of the consultation therefore changes into an exploration of anxiety-management strategies. Clearly this would be linked to the original learning outcomes, but the managing of the patient's anxiety needs to become a primary objective for a time, in order to ultimately fulfil the overall aim. By focusing on the desired outcome, it is easier to objectively assess which methods were successful in moving towards that desired outcome, rather than the intrinsic qualities of skills in themselves. If there are discrepancies between the aims of the two people, then this can be explored as well.

Allow the learner to assess their own performance and to try to think of their own solutions to any problems they encountered. As with Pendleton, this allows the practitioner to analyse their own skills, which is better for their self-esteem as well as providing more robust learning. You should also encourage them to think of alternative strategies to some of the comments made by the group. By encouraging the feedback from the group to be purely descriptive, you can then ask the practitioner to identify the problem and potential ways of dealing with it.

Take suggestions from the rest of the group regarding different strategies that could have been taken. This creates a shared approach to problem-solving that is helpful for both the practitioner and the rest of the group. It also dilutes the effects of positive/negative feedback as it is an approach based far more on problem-solving than on analysis of micro-skills.

Any strategies identified by the practitioner or the group can then be rehearsed and analysed to compare the effectiveness of different strategies. For example:

*Facilitator:* 'OK, Ayesha . . . so how do you feel about that consultation?'
*Practitioner:* 'Well it was OK, I suppose . . .'
*Facilitator:* 'You suppose? Did you have any problems with it then?'
*Practitioner:* 'Well, it started OK . . . but then something went wrong. It

seemed to me like everything was going fine, I was getting on fine with the patient, and then suddenly she seemed to clam up and stop talking to me so openly . . . I just don't know what happened.'

*Facilitator:* 'So, can you think of anything that might have caused that change?'

*Practitioner:* 'Not really . . . I can't think of anything I did . . . I was still maintaining eye contact and stuff . . .'

*Facilitator:* 'Shall we see if your colleagues can help? Did anyone else notice that point in the consultation?'

*Group member 1:* 'Yes . . . I think you had just been asking her about how things had been going at home . . . she had started to tell you about how difficult things had been since her daughter had left.'

*Practitioner:* 'Yes . . . that was it . . . and I asked her how that was making her feel . . .'

*Group member 2:* 'You asked her how that made her feel . . . she was just telling you how worried she was . . . and then you asked her what course her daughter was doing at Sheffield, because your sister is going there next year to do geography . . .'

*Practitioner:* 'That's right . . . she told me but then seemed reluctant to talk about things any more . . .'

*Facilitator:* 'So, what do you think about that Ayesha?'

*Practitioner:* 'Well, perhaps I shouldn't have talked about my sister?'

*Group member 3:* 'I think it would have been OK to talk about your sister, but perhaps not just at that moment, because the patient was just starting to tell you why she was feeling so down . . .'

*Facilitator:* 'So, what else could you have done at that point?'

*Practitioner:* 'Umm . . . I suppose I could have just acknowledged her worries . . .'

*Group member 2:* 'Yeah . . . like you could just have said something like, 'That must be difficult . . .'

*Practitioner:* '. . . yeah . . . or I could have just said nothing . . . and let her talk a bit more about it . . .'

*Facilitator:* 'Shall we see what effect that has on the conversation?'

You can then ask the simulated patient to go back to that part of the consultation and let it run for a few moments with a different intervention, and probably a different outcome.

By doing this, the practitioner has:

➤ identified a problem within the consultation
➤ identified the point at which the problem began
➤ identified which behaviours could have led to the outcome
➤ identified alternative strategies
➤ practised an alternative strategy.

All this has been done with the help of descriptive feedback and suggestions of alternatives from the group, and a little intervention by the facilitator.

It is completely focused on the practitioner's own agenda and goals, and the practitioner and the group members have done all the work themselves.

### A feedback structure based on situational challenge

This is a structure based on the management of a specific challenge or challenges within a consultation. It is a feedback process that takes place throughout the consultation rather than being held at the end, and although the basic principles of feedback apply, beyond that it is very much a reactive process.

It is a useful model to use if you would like to encourage different practitioners to take turns in consulting, as it is a fairly relaxed approach, with the group, rather than the individual practitioner, taking responsibility. As it involves many if not all of the practitioners in the group having a go, it makes it a helpful method to try if your group is made up of nervous practitioners! This may sound like a contradiction – that by expecting all members of the group to have a go, this can be reassuring to the more nervous practitioners. However, as you will see, it is a relaxed collaborative model in which all group members are actively participating all the time, and so it can almost become irrelevant who is in the consulting chair.

Explain that this way of working involves pausing the consultation frequently for discussion, analysis and change of practitioner. The consultation can be paused by anyone in the group, (with the exception of the simulated patient!) and this should be made clear at the beginning of the session.

As you would at the beginning of any stop-start session, you should emphasise that the practitioner who is doing the consultation can take time out at any point and after discussion can either resume the consultation or hand over to someone else.

Again, as with any stop-start session, you should also emphasise that if you, as facilitator, stop the session, it doesn't mean that the practitioner has done anything wrong. This is a wholly interactive process and you will be pausing the consultation frequently in order to encourage this.

You may also say that if anyone in the group has an idea for moving things forward within the consultation, they can also stop the session to make a comment or suggestion or to have a go at implementing their idea.

Clarify with the simulated patient how you would like them to behave during pauses in the consultation. As this process involves frequent pauses in the consultation, it is usually impractical to have the simulated patient running in and out of the room every time it is stopped. However, as it is a process based on management planning, it is not appropriate for the simulated patient to be involved in discussions during the course of the consultation. I would therefore recommend in this kind of session that you ask them to stay in the room but that they freeze, so they are effectively removed from the action. You should also make it clear to the group before the session that, although the simulated patient is physically in the room, they are not a part of the proceedings, and practitioners should pretend that they are not there. The group should act as though the simulated patient cannot hear the discussion, and as such should not feel inhibited about speaking while they are there.

Begin the consultation and stop it fairly soon thereafter. After the initial introductions and a very brief gathering of information about the reason for the interaction you can stop the action. Stopping so early in the interaction may initially seem to make the consultation rather fragmented, but it is important at this stage in the session to establish an atmosphere of relaxed, collaborative work. It can be useful to swap the practitioner at this stage because it really reassures the group that they only need do a tiny part of the consultation. Once they feel more relaxed about having a go, you can leave them to do longer and longer segments, as they are usually perfectly competent, but are simply anxious about 'performing' in front of their peers.

Whenever you pause the consultation, always ask the practitioner how they feel. As you have stopped the action so soon into the consultation they should not have had time to do too much for them to be worried about!

Ask the group what is going on. They should be able to summarise the information gathered so far, or give a reaction to what has happened so far. For example:

> *Practitioner:* 'Hello, Mrs Grandways? My name is Sophie Grant, I'm a staff nurse working on the ward . . . I understand you have some questions you would like answered about your husband's operation?'
>
> *Simulated patient:* 'Well, yes . . . it's just that they told us he would be ready to come home within hours of the operation and now it seems he's going to have to be kept in for another day! I don't understand . . .'
>
> *Facilitator:* 'OK . . . let's stop it there for a moment . . . Sophie, how are you feeling?'
>
> *Practitioner:* 'OK . . .'
>
> *Facilitator:* '. . . tell me what's happened so far . . . all of you . . .'
>
> *Group member:* 'Well, Sophie introduced herself, and they talked about what Mrs Grandways wanted . . .'
>
> *Facilitator:* 'Which is?'
>
> *Group member:* 'Information . . .'
>
> *Facilitator:* 'Yes, information . . . and?'
>
> *Practitioner:* 'Well, she seems a bit upset . . .'
>
> *Group member:* '. . . and confused . . .'
>
> *Facilitator:* 'So, where could we go from here . . .?'

After suggestions, you may want to ask the practitioner if they would like to continue or choose someone else to take over the consultation.

From this point on, just go with the flow! You can stop the consultation whenever you feel it would be useful to do so, and after a while it will feel like such a collaborative process that the group will take control of the exercise themselves!

> One fantastic experience of using this facilitation style I had, was with an inter-professional group, working within the field of paediatrics, who were exploring how to discuss (not break) bad news with parents. Initially apprehensive for all the usual reasons, within about 10 minutes they were jumping in and out of the interviewing chair, trying out different strategies, giving feedback randomly and supportively, and generally forgetting I was there! It doesn't always happen like this, but when it does, it is a brilliant experience of true interactive learning!

Although this style of organising the session does not focus on specific practitioner-based feedback, this should be an element of the process. During discussion, you should highlight strategies and consultation skills used by the practitioners that are effective. You can also, through strategic pausing and discussion, discreetly identify less helpful strategies and explore alternative approaches. This should always be done in a collaborative way, with the group looking for ways of dealing with the presenting challenge, rather than analysing the elements of attempted strategies that were less effective.

At the end, you can ask for feedback from the simulated patient, both in and out of role. It will be unlikely that they can give specific examples, and it is not necessarily appropriate that they do. You can ask them how they were feeling at the beginning of the consultation and how their feelings have changed. You can ask them how satisfied they are with the outcome of the consultation (if there is one!). You can ask them if there were any specific strategies attempted by the practitioners that had an impact on them. They can give more of an insight into the patient's perspective on the consultation, and which management options and consultation strategies were most helpful in the eyes of the patient. You can ask the simulated patient direct questions during the discussion pauses throughout the consultation. However, you must remember always to do this in role and always to keep the questions specific.

This model can be used effectively if you are working with a group looking at particularly challenging consultations or interactions, as the focus is on the particular difficulties presented by the situation. It focuses less on microcommunication skills, rather exploring issues around the management of the interaction. For example:

*Simulated patient:* '*(approaching the practitioner)* I've been sat here for half an hour now . . .'
*Practitioner:* '. . . I'm very sorry, unfortunately the doctor has been . . .'
*Simulated patient:* '. . . you said to me I would be going in after that woman in the corner . . . and now they've called in that other bloke . . .'
*Practitioner:* '. . . well, like I said, the doctor . . .'

*Simulated patient:*   '... it's bloody ridiculous this ... happens every time I come to this bloody practice ... bloody ridiculous ...'

*Practitioner:*   'I'd appreciate it if you'd try not to use that sort of language in here as there are children ...'

*Simulated patient:*   'Don't you tell me about children ... I'll tell you about children ...'

*Facilitator:*   'OK ... let's stop it there ... How are you feeling Brigid?'

*Practitioner:*   'He's scary!'

*Facilitator:*   'Yes ... he's not the happiest man in the world at the moment, is he?! So ... what's happening then?'

*Group member 1:*   'Well, Brigid can't get a word in edgeways ...'

*Group member 2:*   'Yeah, she was trying to be reasonable but he just wasn't letting her ...'

*Group member 3:*   'He's really out of order!'

*Group member 2:*   'She's right to stop him swearing ... we get sick of people thinking they can talk to us any which way they like! It's not on ...'

*Group member 4:*   'Yeah, but it made him even more angry than he was already ...'

The discussion is immediately focused on the problems inherent in the interaction. Practitioners will usually be able to identify the difficulties, and will often spontaneously start to analyse the problems as well as the strategies used to deal with them.

After some discussion, other practitioners may continue the consultation, trying out some of the suggestions made by the group. Further analysis and experimentation with different strategies should lead to a greater understanding of the effects of different communication techniques. As the consultation goes on, the perspective of the simulated patient will become more apparent, creating further understanding on the part of the practitioners as to motivations behind certain behaviours. This should lead to them handling difficult situations more effectively, as they will have more understanding of potential underlying issues.

## WHICH MODEL TO CHOOSE?

The structures you decide to follow and the quality and quantity of feedback that is given will largely depend on the learning outcomes of the session and the make-up of the group you are working with.

The more inexperienced the practitioners, the more structured you will tend to make the feedback. There comes a degree of security around structure and it is a way of, for example, ensuring that the consulting practitioner receives the right blend of positive and constructive feedback to enable them to learn from the experience. As a general rule, you should usually push for a good deal of positive feedback and then when it comes to the points that people feel did not work quite so well, you need to gauge the amount, usually a lot less, that you ask for, depending on the apparent state of mind of the practitioner. However, if the constructive feedback is given in a positive, discursive and supportive way, it is easier to allow for more discussion about these points, as it will naturally become a more generalised approach to exploring the issues.

Also, less experienced practitioners will often need more structure in order to learn and practise the art of giving feedback. It is important that they understand the basic principles, which are often easier to demonstrate within a tighter structure. In this way, it is easier to make it a positive learning experience that builds rather than destroys confidence.

However, if you are working with a group of more confident, experienced practitioners, you will probably tend more towards a less structured, more discursive approach, focusing on problem-solving and management planning rather than micro-communication skills. You may be analysing parts of the consultation, obviously still based on the communication skills of the interviewing practitioner, but more with a view to discussing different strategies and approaches that could be used, and you could reach different outcomes.

We have spoken of the confidence and experience of the practitioners, but in deciding which model would be best to choose, you should also consider your own levels of confidence. It is safer to work within the confines of a firm structure than to have to continually make judgements about where to go with a process. If you are new to the work, you will probably find it easier to begin within the security of a defined structure and gradually you can relax within this to evolve a less rigid process.

Also, some institutions will determine the feedback structure you need to use. There should still be a degree of flexibility within this to keep the process alive, but you basically need to stick to the basic principles as laid down by the institution.

Here is a palette:
➤ Outline the structure for the feedback session, and encourage the group to take ownership of their own learning. I sometimes tell a group that I hope they will take over the session, so that I can have a little snooze in the corner! (Which of course I never do!) At least it gives them the idea that the success of the session depends on their own contributions.
➤ Ask the observing group to take copious notes during the consultation to ensure that everyone is concentrating and has plenty of observations to offer, when asked. Tell them to make their notes as specific and descriptive as possible, writing down the actual words, phrases and gestures used, so that they can give more helpful feedback when they share their observations with the group. Explain that while it is pleasant for a practitioner to hear that they *did really well* or *were really nice*, this doesn't give any lasting guidance to them as to what strategies were effective or which interpersonal skills they should continue to employ.
➤ Ask the observers to divide their page into two halves, on one side noting

the things about the consultation which work well, and on the other those things that could be approached differently.

➤ Decide on the ideal outcome of the situation before the consultation and ask the observers to note down which behaviours contribute to the progress of this and which behaviours hinder it.

➤ Give the observers individual or small-group tasks to undertake during the consultation. For example, one pair could be asked to observe the practitioner's body language, another to note the reactions of the patient, while another could concentrate on the types of questions asked or the use of summaries and so forth.

➤ Ask the practitioner carrying out the consultation whether they have any specific things they would like to receive feedback on, and remind the group of this when they start to share their observations.

➤ Relate the feedback to the desired learning outcomes of the session. For example, the practitioners may be looking at ways to improve the structuring of the consultation, so you could ask the observers to record any examples of structuring techniques such as signposting, or the use of acronyms.

➤ Ask the group to give their feedback directly to the practitioner who has carried out the consultation. This is not always as easy as it sounds, as it is often you, as facilitator, who invites the feedback in the first place and the participants' natural response is to reply to you. If this happens, you can often just look at the interviewing practitioner until the person giving feedback realises. If this fails, sometimes a simple hand gesture will direct the feedback towards the person doing the consultation. If neither of these suggestions work, you may need to gently remind them verbally.

➤ Ask that observations be checked out with the simulated patient (in role) throughout the feedback session. Point out that everyone in the room, apart from the people involved in the interaction, is simply observing. It is only the simulated patient who is on the receiving end of the communication skills demonstrated by the practitioner. This can often open up some interesting discussion about apparent differences in perceptions. By reminding the participants to do this a couple of times, they will soon automatically involve the simulated patient in the discussion. For example:

*Observer:* *(to simulated patient)* 'When the doctor suggested joining a gym, you seemed to get really cross ...?'

*Simulated patient:* 'Well, I'd just like to know where she thinks I'm going to get the money from, to go to a gym!'

*Facilitator:* *(to interviewing practitioner)* 'Can you think of any other ways you could encourage Mrs Williams to take more exercise?'

*Interviewing practitioner:* *(to simulated patient)* 'What if I'd asked you if you had any ideas about how you could take more exercise?'

*Simulated patient:* 'Well . . . I suppose I could walk home from work instead of getting the bus . . . I mean, I would have time for that before the kids get home.'

➤ In this way, you will engender a spontaneous approach to the learning, which is ultimately more enjoyable and more beneficial to the participants as they are more in control of their learning. Also, the more spontaneous you can encourage your group to become, the easier you will find it is to run the session!

➤ You can consciously invite the group to predict how they imagine the simulated patient is feeling about an aspect of the consultation. You would then get the participants to check out the accuracy of the prediction with the simulated patient.

➤ When asking the group for positive feedback, instead of saying:

'Is there anything else you noticed that went well?'

try

'What else did you notice that went well?'

➤ Although this seems like a very minor linguistic alteration, it tends to imply that there are more observations that can be made, and it is up to the group to work harder to find them!

➤ When asking for observations of things that were not quite so effective, you can ask in the same way for a while, and then perhaps alter it to:

'Is there anything else you feel could be tried differently?'

➤ when you feel that the practitioner has had enough suggestions of things that could be changed! I know from observation that practitioners are more likely to opt out of thinking of new things when asked in this way, and so the constructive feedback session can conclude naturally. This is either as a result of the different wording or it is that, as the 'do differentlies' come second in the session, the practitioners are all simply thinking of their lunch/coffee/evening plans!

➤ When a participant makes an observation about something they felt had not worked as well as it might, initially ask them for suggestions as to how they felt it could be improved. Ask the group for their ideas.

➤ Write down your own observations in great detail. You may find it useful to do this even if you are not expecting the observers to write down what they notice, such as if you were using the model based on a situational challenge. In an ideal session, by the end of the consultation, you should have a sheet of observations that you do not need because the practitioner and group have managed to cover all your points! However, if that does not happen you may need to make some comments of your own. Again, remembering that you are facilitating rather than running a didactic teaching session, compare:

*Facilitator:* 'You asked a great open question about Mr Fenwick's symptoms . . . you said, 'Please, can you tell me about your other symptoms' . . . but then you immediately closed it down, by listing what the other symptoms could be . . . you should try to stick to asking the open questions and then leave it up to the patient to respond.'

with

*Facilitator:* 'Can anyone remember how Jane asked Mr Fenwick about his symptoms?'
*Group member 1:* 'She asked an open question . . . 'Can you tell me about your other symptoms?'
*Facilitator:* '. . . mmm . . . and then . . .?'
*Group member 2:* 'Yeah, and then she listed a couple of other symptoms . . . I think it was about his appetite and sleep . . .'
*Facilitator:* 'That's right . . . and what was the response from Mr Fenwick?'
*Interviewing practitioner:* 'Oh, yes . . . he just said he was sleeping OK!'
*Facilitator:* '. . . and what else might you have found out if you had just left a silence after that lovely open question you started with?'
*Interviewing practitioner:* 'I could have found out about his panic attacks right at the beginning.'

The practitioner, with descriptive feedback from the group, has identified a more effective strategy that they may wish to use next time. It may seem more laborious, but this is a far more robust learning experience than simply suggesting to the practitioner your ideas of where they could improve.

During feedback, if alternative strategies are identified, either by the practitioner or by the group, you can invite the practitioner to practise the suggestions. The simulated patient can go back to the relevant point in the consultation, and a brief interaction, focusing on practising the specific alternative suggestions, can provide the opportunity for the practitioner to compare the effectiveness of the suggestion with his/her original strategy. You can also ask the group member who suggested the alternative to come out and try it.

There is huge value for the practitioners in actually rehearsing the suggestions made. However, you must be careful how you facilitate this, as it can seem a little false and disjointed. The practitioners may find it difficult to enter back into the consultation for a short intervention and the simulated patient may feel an obligation to respond positively, however their character really felt.

At the end of the session, you could ask the practitioner who had carried out the consultation to identify one thing they had discovered that they do effectively and one thing that they could think about for the future.

If you have the facilities, it is always worth considering whether or not it is worth recording the feedback as well as the consultation. This gives the practitioner a verbatim account of the observations of their colleagues and the simulated patient. If you do not have recording facilities, it may be worth giving practitioners some form of written feedback. Participants could write down some of their observations at the end of a session if appropriate. A format could be given for this, to give some structure to comments.

## MANAGING THE SIMULATED PATIENT DURING FEEDBACK

As we have seen, feedback can be given in role, out of role or in role neutral and, of course, there are passionate advocators for each method. If we look at the advantages and disadvantages of each, you can assess each learning situation and use whichever seems to be the most appropriate for the particular group and the particular learning objectives.

### In-role feedback

In-role feedback is the feedback given by the simulated patient as the character they have been portraying.

You can ask the simulated patient to give some feedback in role during pauses in a stop-start session. If the group is discussing options or reviewing what has happened in the consultation, you may wish to check whether their assumptions are correct or if the patient has any comments to add.

You can also ask the simulator to give their in-role feedback immediately after the consultation has finished. They will remain as the character they have been playing, and usually in the way they were and felt at the end of the session. You can ask for this feedback, or the practitioner and the observers may ask for it.

#### *Advantages of giving feedback in role*

Advantages include that the feedback is spontaneous and 'from the heart' and that giving feedback in role is a very useful way of the simulated patient giving feedback that may be perceived as negative. They can respond as the character and then temper the criticism when giving more objective feedback out of role. Also, it is perceived as the 'patient's voice' more directly perhaps than feedback given out of role.

#### *Disadvantages of giving feedback in role*

It is sometimes inappropriate for the simulated patient to remain in role after the end of the session, especially if emotions have been high. Also, sometimes the character is not articulate enough to give coherent feedback. It is important that the simulated patient stays in role. They could make a short and simple response, for example:

'Dunno, alright I s'pose.'

There will be time for more constructive comments later, when they are asked to give feedback out of role.

Often the simulated patient may have comments to make from a more 'professional' standpoint. If the practitioner has demonstrated some useful consultation skills, like, for example, techniques like short summaries or signposting (more information about these can be found in Appendix 5), it will be inappropriate for the character to discuss these in such terms. It may be possible for the simulated patient to describe the technique in more casual terms, although this is not always as easy. For example, if they wanted to describe a long summary at the end of a consultation they may be able to say:

> 'When you said about the different things that have been happening to me recently, it really made me feel like you had been listening properly.'

### Out-of-role feedback

Out-of-role feedback is the feedback the simulated patient gives as themselves.

You can ask for feedback from the simulated patient out of role immediately after the consultation, when they could be asked to come out of role as soon as the interaction had ended. In this situation it is not ideal to then expect them to give any in-role feedback.

You may also ask them to give out-of-role feedback immediately after they have given their in-role feedback. Once you have done this, again, it is unfair to ask them for any more in-role feedback.

Sometimes you may decide not to ask them for any out-of role feedback until the end of the session. You may prefer to keep your simulated patients in role during the main feedback discussions if possible. This enables you to check out the assumptions of the group with the patient. It also allows practitioners to practise different approaches and strategies that may be suggested during the feedback discussions.

Once you have asked the simulated patient to come out of role, you may wish to invite them to join in the group discussion about the consultation. This may depend on the situation, time or your perception of the skills of the simulated patient.

### *Advantages of giving feedback out of role*

Simulated patients are able to explain comments that they may have made during feedback given in role. This may make possibly negative comments more constructive. For example, in role their feedback could highlight a potential lack of empathy by saying:

> 'She was a right stuck-up cow . . . she didn't give a monkey's for how I was going to get home.'

This would have raised the issue of empathy but maybe not in the most constructive form! In their out-of-role feedback, they are able to lessen the impact of the negative comment (which has been heard) by saying something like:

> 'I think it must be very difficult for anyone to warm to Pat . . . she is such an aggressive sort of person. I just wondered, perhaps, if you had been able to show a bit more interest in her plight, you may have been able to reach the person beneath the hard exterior.'

The simulated patients are able to use different vocabulary, maybe enabling some points to be made more clearly. They should not, for example, use communication skills jargon while still in role, but it is often easier to give feedback concisely by using descriptive terminology with examples.

They can refer to their own experience (being careful not to breach confidentiality!), although it is important to encourage them to keep this relevant. It is important that they remain focused on the task in hand and on their role as a learning resource. Simulated patients who talk too much about their own lives often distract from the main teaching aims.

They are not constrained by the mood or attitudes of the character they have been playing.

They are able to draw on their own knowledge of the character they have been playing from a more objective stance.

> I remember one character I played for a number of years who was very aggressive and threatening. The consultations usually focused on how to deal with her without getting hurt (not that we ever really hurt people!) and without giving in to her demands. She was pregnant and I vividly remember one medical student who ignored all the demands and threats, and focused instead on how the patient was feeling about the proposed abortion. After a while the session was paused and I left the room to allow them to explore different strategies. While I was waiting to be called back in, I found there were tears rolling down my cheeks. I suddenly had a real understanding of how vulnerable this character was if anyone reached through her tough exterior. This gave me a much deeper knowledge of this character and although this would rarely be able to be expressed in role, it meant that I could give more insight into her character in my out-of-role feedback.

### Disadvantages of giving feedback out of role
Disadvantages include feedback being less immediate and that the simulated patient is drawn away from the intensity of the experience. It is often easier to talk about something than to experience it, yet it is often in the experiencing of it that the most powerful learning takes place.

## Role-neutral feedback

Role-neutral feedback is simply feedback from the character without the strong emotions that may have been evident during the consultation. It is a subtle and sophisticated technique, which involves the simulated patient imagining their character in a less emotionally charged situation.

Role neutral is useful in as much as it can have some of the advantages of both in-role feedback and out-of-role feedback. However, it does also dilute some of the positive effects of both.

### *Advantages of giving feedback in role neutral*

Advantages include that the simulated patient is able to maintain some of the spontaneity of in-role feedback while giving more objective feedback and they are able to give feedback in role without continuing the consultation with all the emotions that may have been present. Also, they are able to give more information about the patient's life as they will not be constrained by the attitudes and moods of the patient in the scenario.

### *Disadvantages of giving feedback in role neutral*

Disadvantages include that it is not always an easy thing to do to remain in character yet without the emotions of the current situation. You therefore need an experienced simulated patient who is confident in this practice. Also, if the character is near to the simulated patient's own personality, it can be unclear whether their feedback is in role or out of role. It is easy for the simulator to become confused and begin to give in-role or out-of-role feedback.

You will need to choose what feedback method would be best depending on the nature of the character, the scenario, the group and on what happened during the consultation. Allowing the simulated patient to give both in-role and out-of-role feedback is usually the most useful option, if this is possible. The most important thing about the great 'in-role/out-of-role' debate is that the simulated patient should ideally be given the opportunity to give feedback both in role and out of role.

If a simulator knows that they will definitely be given the chance to give some feedback out of role, they will be less likely to compromise their role by giving inappropriate feedback in role. You should always clarify your intentions about this with the simulated patient at the beginning of the session, as it can be very frustrating for them not to be given the chance to give some feedback out of role and effectively to debrief.

It is important to make it very clear to the simulated patient when you want them to be in role and out of role. They should remain in role until you direct them otherwise, and it is as well to clarify this with them before the session. During the session, you can make it clearer by addressing them by their character name if you want them to give feedback in role, and by their real name if you want them to be out of role. When out of role, it is useful if you talk about the character in the third person. For example:

> *Facilitator:* *(to simulated patient in role)* 'Mrs Webster, can you tell us how it felt for you when the doctor told you that you would need to go into hospital?'

> *Facilitator:* *(to simulated patient out of role)* 'Janine . . . could you give us an idea why Mrs Webster was so upset when the doctor mentioned the possibility of going into hospital?'

This makes it very clear to both the simulated patient and the group whether they are talking to the simulated patient in or out of role.

It is important to make sure the group are aware of whether the simulated patient is still in role during feedback, and to make it clear when you are asking them to come out of role. You can introduce them to the group by their real name and then ask them if they have anything else they would like to comment on about the process, out of role.

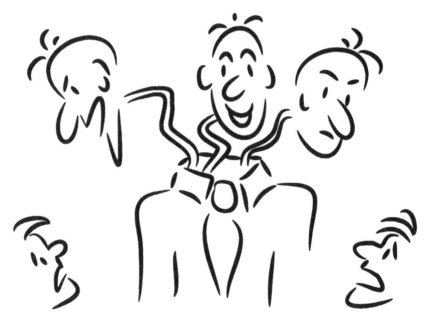

**'Don't worry . . . it's only the simulated patient's new feedback technique!'**

## THINGS TO ENCOURAGE OR TO GIVE FEEDBACK ON

As I mentioned earlier, unless you are a super-confident facilitator, I think it is always a good idea to write down your own observations during the course of the consultations. Although you should be able to encourage the group to produce most of the comments, it is useful to have noted down any salient points just in case no one else has picked them up. It also gives you more confidence to encourage the group to give more feedback if you have identified other things to say yourself.

There are many things listed in Chapter 4 that you, as well as the simulated patient, may choose to give feedback on. In addition, the following suggestions may be easier for observers to note rather than the simulated patient, as they are technique based or process based rather than feeling based.

➤ Did the introduction cover the necessary details? Did the practitioner check the patient's name and date of birth?

➤ Did they clarify how the patient would like to be addressed?

➤ Did they give their own name and role within the organisation and the consultation?

➤ Did the practitioner clarify the reason for the interaction?

➤ Was consent obtained? Was it informed consent? Did the practitioner outline the purpose of the interaction?

➤ Was confidentiality discussed appropriately and accurately, with a view to who, realistically, may be involved in the patient's care?

➤ You will possibly have discussed the seating arrangements before the consultation begins, but it may be worth getting feedback from the simulated patient about how successful the agreed plan was.

➤ You may also want to discuss the use of the computer/notes during a consultation, if this could not be explored because of logistic reasons.

➤ How did the seating arrangement facilitate the focus on the patient when there was a relative, friend or interpreter in the room?

➤ What techniques did the practitioner use to build a rapport with the patient?

➤ Did they use appropriate language or did they hide behind medical jargon?

➤ What skills of active listening did they demonstrate?

➤ How did they show empathy – through comments, expression, touch, use of silence?

➤ Were sensitive techniques used to cope with emotions displayed during the consultation? Posture? Voice? Appropriate language?

➤ In what ways did the practitioner demonstrate professionalism?

➤ Were there any opportunities for professional integrity to be shown?

➤ What attempts were made to structure the consultation – overall structure, use of acronyms, notes and so forth? How successful were they?

➤ Was the practitioner able to weave the structure into the patient's own story or did it seem as though they were completing a checklist?

➤ Did the practitioner use signposting to make it clear to the patient what they were going to talk about and why? Was consent gained appropriately?

➤ Was summarising used effectively to maintain clarity throughout the consultation and ensure that information exchanged was accurate?

➤ Was a patient-centred approach used to take a history, or was it practitioner led?

➤ Was enough time left for the patient to tell their story? Were listening skills used effectively to encourage this?

➤ Were short summaries and silences used to encourage the patient to give further information?

➤ Did the practitioner negotiate effectively with the patient or were they prescriptive or paternalistic in their approach?

➤ Were open and closed questions used to good effect?

➤ Did the practitioner ask any leading questions?

➤ Were there any times when they asked multiple questions, which led to some information being lost because the patient only answered the first or last question?

➤ When the consultation moved on to developing a management plan, did the practitioner involve the patient in this discussion, or did they simply tell them what was going to happen?

➤ Were options explored with the patient?

➤ Did the practitioner take into account the patient's own concerns and expectations when discussing what could happen next?

➤ When information was given was it given clearly?

➤ What methods were used to make it easier for the patient to understand – rephrasing, diagrams, hand gestures, leaflets and so forth?

➤ How did the practitioner ensure that the patient had understood the information given? Did they chunk the information appropriately and then ask if the patient had understood each stage?

➤ Asking questions? Summarising? Asking the patient to summarise?

➤ Were there any particularly difficult or significant moments in the consultation that the practitioner handled sensitively and effectively?

➤ Was the practitioner able to pick up on verbal and non-verbal clues during the consultation?

# CHAPTER 12

# Any other business!

## KEEPING PEOPLE SAFE

It is your job as facilitator to keep all the people involved in the session safe. There should be no physical risks involved, although it is occasionally helpful to remind the participants of this, especially if you are running a workshop on managing aggression!

> As part of a conference about managing conflict, just before lunch, there was a presentation by the police force on self-defence. After lunch there were to be two simulated patient sessions, where delegates could explore different ways of managing potentially volatile situations. During the first of these, one overenthusiastic delegate decided to practise some of the techniques of takedown demonstrated by the police in the morning on the poor, pretending-to-be-aggressive simulated patient! Since then, I will often make a point of promising that, however angry they may seem, the simulated patients will not hurt the practitioners and politely ask that they may show the simulated patients the same respect!

However, keeping people safe within the session refers more to emotional safety. Sometimes, as with all forms of creative work, people can be deeply, and often quite unexpectedly, affected by some of the issues explored. It may be advisable to offer a health warning to the group at the beginning of the session.

If you are working on a breaking bad news scenario, it is fairly obvious that you need to mention to the group that the sensitive subject matter may make the session quite difficult for some people, if, for example, they have experienced similar trauma in their own lives. However, you should also be aware of the sessions that seem quite straightforward and unemotional, because sometimes we can be surprised by the pathway that the consultation takes, and how different experiences can affect people in different ways. Simulated patient work is rarely predictable! As you are always working with human emotions, you will find that people can become upset by seemingly benign interactions. It is often worth just mentioning this, therefore, if you feel there is a chance of any emotional

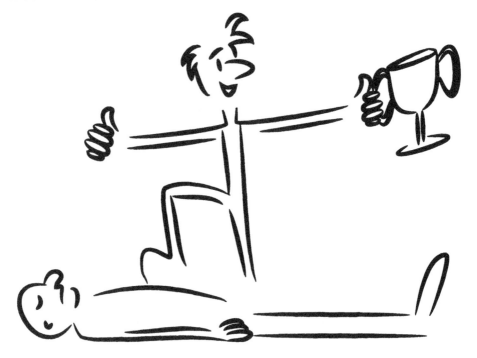

**'And the fourth round goes to Dr. Verbera!'**

challenges arising, in order to enable people to prepare to take care of themselves if necessary.

You will need to decide how you would like any distress to be handled. It may be best that practitioners are simply able to leave the room if needs be, with or without a colleague. It may be preferable to encourage the practitioners to stay in the room and offer each other support within the session. Opinions differ on this, as some facilitators believe that such situations may occur in practice and therefore it is better to learn how to handle them in a safe and supportive environment. Others feel that it is not a therapy group and such support within the session would be too disruptive to the designated learning objectives of the session. Whichever way you decide to deal with such a situation, if it arises, you should always personally make sure that people are feeling all right at the end of the session, both as a group and individually if necessary.

Apart from obviously emotionally challenging scenarios, you should also keep people safe from potentially damaging feedback. You should try to avert this from the beginning by being clear with the group about the expected quality of feedback. You should also try to monitor this during the session and limit the effects of potentially upsetting feedback by discussion or diversion. It is sometimes necessary to speak with a practitioner who has received some difficult feedback at the end of the session. Make sure that they have heard the positive feedback, that they have been able to take the constructive feedback in a way that is helpful and that they do not feel completely demoralised by it.

## CLOSING THE SESSION

Often discussions during and after simulated patient sessions can be extensive, if there are really interesting issues to explore. However, it is good practice to allow a short space of time at the end to close the session. This is important to enable you to make sure everyone is feeling positive and ready to return to the un-simulated world, and also to summarise the learning that has taken place for the group. This gives you an opportunity to talk about any issues that may remain unresolved from the discussions or from the exercises.

You may use the time to make sure everyone feels comfortable with the feedback they have received, or with the issues that have been discussed. If the session has been challenging, it will give you the opportunity to make sure that everyone can view it as a positive experience, and that they can appreciate the value of what they have learnt, however difficult it may have been.

If you discussed or developed learning objectives at the beginning of the session, you should allow time to revisit them to see whether the group feel they have been fulfilled. This is especially important if the participants have identified their own personal learning objectives. This also helps to consolidate the learning outcomes of the session.

You may wish to do some kind of closing exercise, perhaps identifying what learning the practitioners feel they have gained from the session. You may, for example, ask the practitioners to identify something they have learnt from the session in general. You may ask each practitioner for something positive they have learnt about their practice and something they will work on for the future. In keeping with the emphasis in feedback, you may ask each practitioner for two positive things they have learnt about their practice and one that they will think about developing. One endearing way this can be described is to ask for two stars and a wish! These can be written down and kept by the participants.

You may ask the practitioners to think about what changes they may wish to introduce into their workplace as a result of the session – for example, around safety issues or interprofessional communication issues.

Another good way of reinforcing the learning can be to ask them to write their thoughts on a self-addressed postcard. These can then be sent to them at a specified number of weeks after the session. This enables them to remind themselves of the issues explored in the session and of their own learning. They can also evaluate whether the learning has allowed them to implement any changes to their working practice or environment. If you are able to have a follow-up session, this can also act as an evaluation for the longer-term effectiveness of the session.

## EVALUATION

You may wish to evaluate the session in some way. Some kind of standard evaluation may be already established within the organisation you are working for, but if not you may decide that some kind of review of the session would be worthwhile. This is useful for your own professional development and also for development of simulated patient work in the future.

You could simply do it in an informal way by discussion with the group of practitioners you have been working with. You will have to genuinely encourage them to be honest in their feedback both of the session and of you as facilitator. You may actually need to ask them which specific parts they found less or more helpful.

You could devise a written evaluation sheet to be completed at the end of the session/s. This could be in the form of boxes to tick or, more usefully, it could include space to write specifically which parts of the session were effective and if there were any suggestions for improvements in the future.

As previously mentioned, you should always try to take the opportunity to ask the simulated patient how they felt the session had gone and if they had any observations to make about how to improve it. Often simulated patients work for many different organisations and will automatically compare and contrast different styles of working. As observed previously, they may need some encouragement to be frank about difficult issues, but if you can get honest feedback from your simulated patients, it can be extremely valuable.

## TROUBLESHOOTING

As with any interactive process involving those unpredictable creatures human beings, there is the potential for a vast number of unexpected challenges! While you must understand that this is to some extent the nature of the beast (and what makes it such an exciting way to work!), it may be useful to consider some of the potential pitfalls before you begin so you can put into place some strategies to deal with these challenges.

Sometimes practitioners may feel that they are already effective communicators and are reluctant to engage in an exercise they feel to be superfluous to their needs.

It may be helpful to point out that while they may have fantastic interpersonal skills, managing a consultation effectively or dealing with a particularly challenging situation professionally are more specific skills that may often benefit from a little attention. Just as someone may be a gifted sportsperson, it takes practice and training to develop them into a professional; so it is with consultation skills.

Sometimes practitioners may complain that the situation is artificial. This can be general; for example, a medical student may argue:

> 'This is nothing like taking a history on the ward . . . I can do it on the
> ward but I can't do it with everyone watching.'

In this case, you could emphasise that the aim of the exercise is not to reproduce a real-life situation. Rather, you are working together to create an opportunity to explore and practise different approaches to communication, and to identify micro-skills we can develop to improve our consultation style. Often, students and sometimes even qualified practitioners will make such complaints in an attempt to disguise their nervousness or perceived lack of skill. It is important to clarify the value of the work to the practitioners, but also to reassure the participants about the supportive and non-threatening nature of the group.

Sometimes the complaints are more specific to a place of work and working procedures. For example, a receptionist may say:

> 'That could never happen here because the nurse practitioner would always be available to see that patient.'

Again, you could make it clear that this is a learning situation and not a faithful reproduction of real life. You could emphasise the fact that the skills you are practising are transferable and so have value in a number of different situations.

If complaints were that a scenario or character was unrealistic, you could point out that all the scenarios are based on real cases (although only if they are, obviously!).

Never underestimate the power of humour and self-parody! Imagine, for example, that you are working with a scenario for receptionists, and you want them to work with it rather than passing the buck to the medical staff or the practice manager, as they may perfectly legitimately do in their practice. You could perhaps cite the dreadful lurgy that has laid half the doctors off, with all other staff at a conference/on holiday/at the dentist's/watching their child's nativity play . . . In this way, you are emphasising the artificiality of the situation, but in a humorous way so that you are not only making them less likely to shy from the challenge but also you are building a more relaxed atmosphere.

Sometimes you may find yourself in a situation where a simulated patient gets a little carried away and gives what they clearly feel is an Oscar-winning performance, but which is, nonetheless, not helpful in providing a suitable environment to enable the group to reach their learning outcomes.

The best way to deal with this is through sensitive communication with the simulated patient, although this can be difficult! Some thespians can be very touchy if they feel that their acting talents are criticised! Alternatively, you can deal with the consultation as it is, and then discuss any problems it may have caused, with the group, after the simulated patient has left.

Sometimes despite your best efforts at explaining the importance of sensitive feedback, you may encounter the situation where some group members, or indeed the simulated patients themselves, are giving somewhat destructive feedback. One effective way to deal with this situation, rather than directly drawing attention to the difficulty, is to summarise what the person is saying with a positive connotation to it. For example, if a group member says:

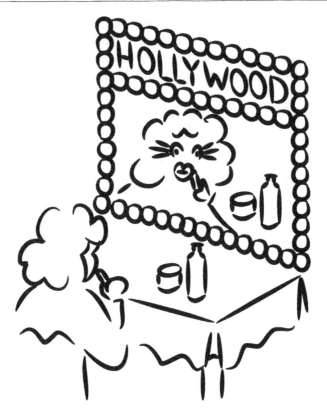

**The simulated patients' dressing room!**

> 'You seemed really cold in the way you were just asking question after question, you didn't take any notice of how she was feeling even when she was clearly upset about the questions you were asking.'

you could say:

> 'So what you're saying is that you felt that there may have been places in the conversation when Mark could have focused on the patient's concerns, without perhaps losing the excellent structure he had created?'

You could then ask the consulting practitioner to think about any places when they could have shown empathy, and how they could have done it. If they are not sure, the rest of the group can be invited to suggest some. In this way, you are taking the focus of the feedback away from the practitioner and moving it to the consultation and techniques of showing empathy. You are also allowing the consulting practitioner to identify the solutions to the difficulty. A few examples of positive connotation from you should be enough to guide the group back to giving more sensitive constructive feedback.

Occasionally, you may find a simulated patient talking inappropriately about their own experiences, sometimes completely unrelated to anything that has occurred during the session. This is another delicate situation that needs to be dealt with using tact and diplomacy. When you ask the simulated patient to come out of role at the end, it is sometimes helpful to specify exactly what kind of comments you are looking for. If you don't want the group entertained by anecdotes about the time the simulated patient trekked across the Sahara on a camel with a broken leg, you could try asking them specifically if they have anything else to add '*about the process*'. In this way it should be clear that they should really be giving feedback on the session and not sharing their life story. If, despite this tactic, they still insist on launching into a tale, you can use body language – perhaps gathering your papers and sitting on the edge of your seat – to try to hint that it is time to move on. You may be able to discuss this with the simulated patient after the session, depending on the sophistication of your skills of diplomacy!

You may find yourself facing a group of 'treacle waders'. If all your attempts at warming them up and relaxing them fail, then it is often a good idea to become more directive. Specific feedback tasks can be given to individuals, 'volunteers' can be chosen . . . (you can either do this directly or you can number a group list and then get someone to choose a number) and questions can be asked directly. It may also be worth laying your cards on the table. Bring it to their attention that the session will not function without their participation, and the more enthusiastic their participation, the more enjoyable the session will be for everyone.

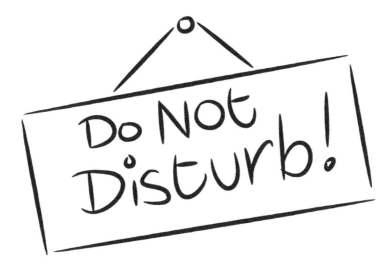

**'This is not an option!'**

Obviously, the kinds of problems you may face will be as varied as the kinds of groups and the kinds of people you will be working with, so I can't give you a comprehensive list of complaints and remedies!

One of my favourite ways of approaching any difficulties that arise is by redefining them as 'interesting challenges'! This may seem like pedantic wordplay, but the technique is common and effective . . . dynamic family therapy calls it positive connotation, permaculture states that the problem is the solution and in t'ai chi the force is not resisted but yielded to and worked with! If you can approach any problems that arise in your sessions in this way, as well as asking for support and help from your colleagues, then you will soon gain in confidence and establish a repertoire of tactics for dealing with challenges that suit you and your way of working.

# PART FOUR

# Assessment and other uses of simulated patients

*For everything you have missed, you have gained something else, and for everything you gain, you lose something else.*
Ralph Waldo Emerson (1803–1882)

# CHAPTER 13

# Standardised patients in examinations and recruitment interviews

Standardised patients can be used in the assessment of health professionals in a variety of different ways; indeed, examinations form a large part of the work available to simulated patients. They tend to be called standardised patients when working in an assessment situation, as this reflects the slightly different emphasis for the work. I will describe some of the more common uses of simulators that are in current practice.

## EXAMINATIONS

In recent years, it has been increasingly appreciated how much simulated patients can contribute to the examination process both within undergraduate healthcare settings and for qualified professionals as they progress up the career ladder.

As healthcare education becomes more sophisticated, there is greater integration of clinical and interpersonal skills. This is a very positive move since research has shown that the quality of interpersonal communication throughout a person's healthcare experience can have a profound effect on their clinical outcomes. However, currently there are three types of examination challenges that affect the use of simulated patients: the clinical skills examination, the consultation skills examination and the examination that is a combination of both. The examination that tests a candidate's clinical expertise may or may not involve an element of communication skills assessment.

### Clinical skills examinations

If the assessment contains no element of interpersonal skills, it is more likely that the physical examination is carried out on a healthy volunteer or on a mannequin.

A healthy volunteer is a volunteer patient or student who allows the candidate to examine them or carry out some non-invasive clinical procedure, in return for expenses or a small fee. This is much cheaper than using a simulated patient. Low-fidelity mannequins are used commonly for more invasive procedures.

### Consultation skills stations

Some stations are designed to test a candidate's consultation skills alone. These may include basic skills of history taking or explaining a procedure to a patient, or they may be assessing more complex specialist skills, such as breaking bad news or negotiating a treatment plan with a reluctant patient.

Sometimes candidates are expected to deal with strong emotions such as anger or grief, or assess a mental health problem. Often, the roles given to the simulated patient for exams are reasonably straightforward, although this will not always be the case. Generally speaking, the more qualified the candidate, the more complex the role will be. This may be on the level of clinical detail, social situation or psychological and emotional responses.

The simulated patients should have received additional training for the role they are playing (*see* Chapter 4), although this is sometimes less comprehensive than it should be. Therefore, it is essential that you allow time before the examination begins to talk with your simulated patient about the role, the situation and the expectations of the candidate. If there are any issues arising from this that could affect consistency or validation, it is vital that you address them with the other simulated patients and the examining body.

Sometimes, although the main purpose of the station is to assess a candidate's communication skills, they may need to perform an examination during the course of the consultation. There are three options in this case.

First, if it is a non-invasive procedure, the standardised patient may be happy simply to undergo the examination. In this case, you would need to ensure that the standardised patient had no abnormal signs that would affect the examination. For example, if the candidate were to do a peak flow test which showed poor results, they may assume the character was suffering with asthma when in fact it was the standardised patient's own problem!

You should also check that the standardised patient actually feels that the procedure is non-invasive. Some simulators are happy to have their breasts examined while others find an examination of their throat, when they are well, uncomfortable! You should also bear in mind that while one abdominal examination may be harmless enough, twenty-one abdominal examinations by inexperienced practitioners may not be! It is important to make sure that the standardised patient understands exactly what the examination entails, and is happy to go ahead with it.

> The most pleasant examination I have undergone was when I was playing the part of a woman who needed a lymph node investigation. The main examination procedure seemed to involve a gentle massage of my neck and shoulder area. After a dozen or so candidates, I found myself drifting off into an extremely relaxed state, and was sorry when the gong sounded to announce the end of the examination!

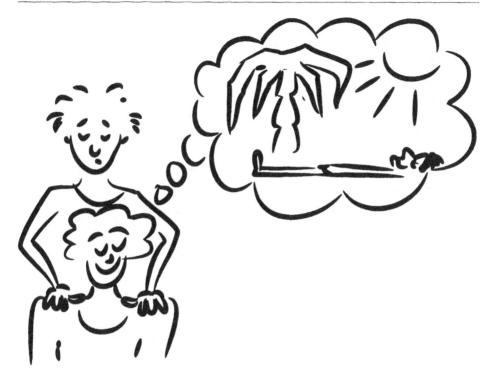

**'Hmmmmm . . .!'**

However, you have to take the rough with the smooth in this work . . . the most uncomfortable examination I have undergone was when students were asked to test for sensation loss in my legs. The way they were expected to do this was by sticking pins in both legs, and I was to tell them when I felt anything. Unfortunately, as I was supposed to have lost all feeling in my left leg, I therefore could not react in any way to the pain! Not quite so pleasant!

Second, you may give a card to the standardised patient to hand to the candidate at the appropriate time. Sometimes the standardised patient is issued with more than one card to present to the candidate containing the findings of different examinations. You should remind them before the examination that they should keep them in separate places and only give each one in response to the relevant and specific question. They should remember where they have put each one, as it is not good for the simulated patient to inadvertently indicate to the student that there are further investigations that they should be carrying out, by producing more than one card or the wrong one.

Third, you can interrupt when a candidate says they would like to examine the patient, ask them to specify exactly which examinations they would carry out and give them the results.

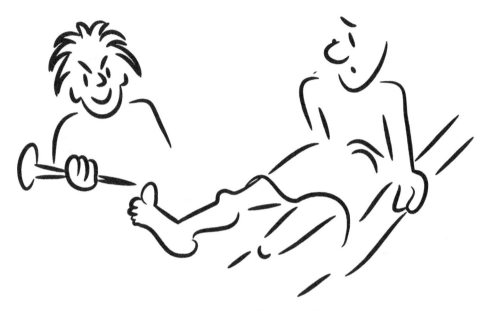

**'Just tell me if you can feel anything touching your foot . . .!'**

### Integrated stations

There is an increasing tendency to use integrated stations in examinations as these provide a more realistic assessment of the candidates' skills.

#### Dealing with the integrated station

Low-fidelity part-body mannequins are often used to provide the 'body' in an integrated station. This is a useful method when the candidate is expected to demonstrate an invasive procedure or when the candidate is expected to discover some abnormal pathology.

This may mean, for example, that a candidate is expected to catheterise a lower-body mannequin that is attached to a standardised patient playing an anxious person who needs reassurance throughout the procedure. It may mean that a standardised patient is wearing prosthetic breasts to enable the discovery of a lump. The candidate is expected not only to find and identify the lump but also to deal with the patient's anxieties while carrying out the examination. High-fidelity mannequins can also be voiced-over by a standardised patient.

Standardised patients can be trained to accurately portray many physical signs. Although it would seem fairly limited, in fact there are a huge number of conditions that can be accurately represented. The key to the success of this is thorough training of the simulated patient and sufficiently detailed information in their brief. In the case of a shoulder injury, for example, the standardised patient can be trained to display the exact amount and type of pain, mobility (abduction, adduction, rotation and so forth), and physical posture to enable the candidate to make an accurate diagnosis. This can be aided by the subtle use of make-up to provide inflammation, bruising and so forth. This is a more realistic and therefore a more effective way of examination, although obviously limited by the invasiveness of procedures and an absence of pathology.

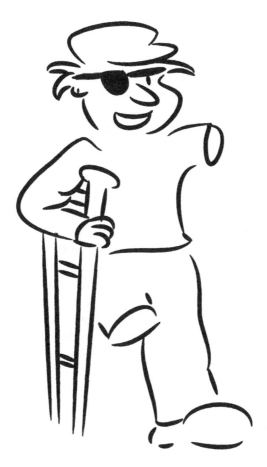

**'This is my fourth OSCE . . . wonder what scenario I'll get this time!'**

You may find yourself in the position of being an examiner in an examination station that has a simulated patient as part of the 'equipment' (as I mentioned previously, simulated patients can feel quite bemused when they find themselves listed between the stopwatch and the peak flow meter as equipment!). Obviously in all decisions and actions you must be guided by the instructions and rules of the examining body. However, as there is a greater potential for the unexpected in standardised patient stations, there are a few things specific to the nature of this kind of assessment that you may wish to consider.

As much as time permits, talk with your standardised patient before the examination begins. You should check that the simulator has adequate information and is clear about the information that they have. Specifically, you should make sure that their clinical information, both physical and psychological, is accurate and complete, and that any relevant social elements are clear.

It may be worth discussing the pace at which the information should be delivered. Standardised patients should be trained to 'chunk' the information, but it is probably a good idea to briefly discuss this or at least remind them of this before they begin.

You may also like to talk with them about your expectations as regards how you are expecting the information to be elicited. The standardised patient must endeavour to give the same information to each candidate. This may not sound too difficult, but when questions are posed differently by different candidates, it is not always easy to work out which piece of information they have asked for. If a candidate asks a series of open questions, backed up with effective verbal and non-verbal encouragement, they should be rewarded for this as much as the candidate who asks a series of closed questions about symptoms should receive direct answers to their direct questions. This is a challenging area and requires the standardised patient to make judgements throughout the consultation. You should bear in mind the complexity of this task if you feel surprised at a standardised patient's response within a consultation. If there is an opportunity, you could discuss such incidents between stations or at the break.

I find it useful to share with the standardised patient the sort of information I am looking for within a station. This may involve briefly going through the marking sheet so that they know, for example, if there is a counselling element, or whether the candidate is expected to ask about social history. This is not to encourage him/her to help the student in any way, but will enable them to make responses to irrelevant questions brief, so as to allow the candidate time to focus on the main issues.

If there are any omissions in the information given to the simulated patient, you may need to give them the additional information. If there are several stations with the same scenario, it is crucial that you convey this additional information to the other simulators and examiners, to ensure consistency. You should also note the changes to report back to the examining authorities afterwards.

You should check that the information given to the standardised patient corresponds with your marking sheet. Any discrepancies may be obvious as you read through the material, but sometimes they don't become evident until the first candidate embarks on their interview. Whether you make small changes to the role, the marking sheet, or leave it as it is and simply note the difficulty as feedback will depend mainly on the rules of the examining body, but may also be influenced by time and the nature of the difficulties presented.

You should also check that there is correlation between the simulated patient's information, the examiner's information and the candidate's information which is given outside and inside the station. It can be quite disconcerting for all concerned if a candidate enters expecting to talk about a mother's 15-year-old son only to find she is worried about her 10-year-old daughter!

Sometimes the standardised patient may impede the success of the station because of their interpretation of the role. It is the job of the standardised patient to provide the candidate with the opportunity to demonstrate their skills and knowledge. If for any reason they are not doing this, you may need to address the issue, depending on the nature and severity of the problem. Again, your way of dealing with this situation will depend on many external factors, but if it is allowed and you have the opportunity, it can be worth offering a little guidance after the first candidate.

Finally, it can be a gruelling process! Ensure you have water, pens and other necessary equipment for yourself, your standardised patient and your candidates!

### Recruitment interviews

Another way in which simulated patients can be used in an assessment situation is in the recruitment process. An individual general practice surgery may wish to recruit a new practice manager, a deanery may seek new trainees for a general practitioner or specialist rotation, or a department within a hospital may be seeking new consultants or managers. The basic principles of recruitment are similar to those for examinations, as the process should come under similar scrutiny and prove similarly robust.

You may decide to give your standardised patients actual key phrases to include in the consultation, in order to promote consistency. For example, you may ask them to start with the opening phrase:

'I can't believe it's taken so long for me to get this referral through!'

This ensures that the same tone is set at the beginning to achieve greater consistency, especially if you are using more than one standardised patient. Although there will always be slight differences in approach, all the simulators should be demonstrating similar levels of frustration as they walk through the door.

There may be set key phrases, to be used verbatim or creatively, that the standardised patient is to use during the consultation. These can help them to express certain emotions, such as confusion or fear. This should then provide each candidate with the same opportunity to demonstrate core competencies, such as ability to cope under pressure, empathy and professional integrity. This can be challenging for the standardised patients, but is effective in maintaining a consistent environment in which to assess the candidates.

Ideally, the standardised patients should be offered training if there is more than one at a recruitment event. You may ask the standardised patients, as with examinations, to give feedback or to score the candidate. You should, again, give them clear guidance as to how this will happen and what is expected.

Working as a standardised patient within an examination or recruitment setting differs considerably from the role of the simulated patient within a teaching session. In the teaching session they need to be far more reactive, responding to communication strategies employed by the practitioner and observing how they feel about different techniques. They should also be doing this, to a large extent, within an examination or recruitment situation, but they may need to be more in the driving seat of the consultation than they are required to be in teaching sessions. They must still be essentially reactive, but may also need to be proactive in moving the session on at times, as you, as examiner, are not there to facilitate the situation but to observe it. It helps to make the standardised patients aware of this extra responsibility.

If, for example, a candidate is insensitive about something during the consultation, the standardised patient should indicate their distress in some way to give the candidate a chance to rectify the situation, but should then move on. You can note the lack of sensitivity, but if the simulator does not shift the focus, the candidate will not have the opportunity to display other skills. If a similar difficulty were to arise during a teaching session, you would be facilitating and could therefore manage the situation, but in an exam you must allow and encourage the simulator to take responsibility for creating the necessary opportunities for the candidates to demonstrate their skills.

The interview may take the format of an examination with different stations. However, it is more likely that the interaction with a simulated patient/relative/colleague will be only one part of the process, with additional group exercises, written exercises, multiple-choice questionnaires and one-to-one interviews.

The simulated patient interaction may take place in a room with the candidate, examiner and standardised patient present, or it may be recorded in one room, with a video link to another room where it is observed by a panel of examiners. The benefit of this is that the examiners can discuss the proceedings and also that the interaction is recorded, which may be useful if there were to be any subsequent challenges to the process.

It also provides a resource for standardisation, should the process need to be repeated with different simulated patients.

### Examination/recruitment preparation courses

There are many courses offered that allow practitioners to practise the skills needed to pass examinations. They are often for high-level qualifications such as registration as general practitioners or hospital consultants, and they offer the chance to explore the assessment format in a theoretical way as well as giving the opportunity to practise the type of stations that will be used in the actual examination.

The way in which simulated patients are used in these sessions is a cross between the way they are used in examinations and teaching sessions. The format imitates the examination format, with a number of different stations testing the candidates' skills. However, unlike in an examination, you can ask the simulated patient to offer feedback to the candidates afterwards. Usually you will be giving feedback with the simulator, but occasionally you can ask them to give feedback on their own, depending on the nature of the station and the feedback required.

Their feedback may be general consultation skills feedback, or you may ask them to give feedback on specific examination techniques. Receiving such guidance can stand the candidates in much better stead when they face the actual assessment.

This section outlines a few pointers you may wish to give the candidates in your examination/recruitment preparation sessions.

As in all examinations, emphasise the importance of reading the question. If a question asks that they take a focused history, they should not waste time taking a full history. If a question asks that they explain their findings to the patient, they should not explain them to the examiner.

Remind them that the standardised patient is actually a part of the question, not simply a passive model for them to demonstrate their skills on. Simulators form a very active part of the assessment, and as such, all information given by them should be relevant. The standardised patients are trained to give the candidates information that is significant, provided it is asked for in an appropriate manner. You should tell the practitioners to observe the simulators closely throughout the consultation, watching closely for any non-verbal communication as well as all aspects of their verbal comments. Here are a couple of examples of how the standardised patient's behaviour may form part of the question:

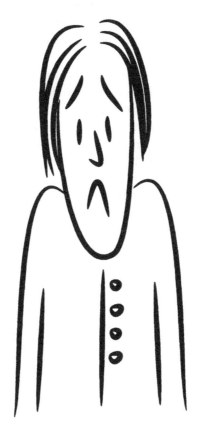

'I'm fine, thank you . . .'

> *Candidate:* 'So, tell me . . . how do you find you are coping with the baby?
> *Standardised patient:* Oh, fine . . . she smiled at me yesterday.'

The standardised patient may speak these words in an animated tone, maintaining eye contact with the candidate and smiling. However, she may say exactly the same words, but she may look down, sigh and sound very flat. It is alarming how many candidates will ignore these overt signals, and then in defence of their failure will say:

> 'But she said everything was fine, she talked about the baby smiling!'

In another station, a candidate may be confronted with a seemingly angry patient.

> *Standardised patient:* 'Well, I was so cross . . . that doctor who referred me on here . . . well, I don't think he had a clue what he was on about . . . seemed to be glad to get rid of me . . . you should do something about these locums.'

The standardised patient may be angry, but they may not simply be moaning about the last doctor they saw because they are in a bad mood! They may well be indicating to the candidate that their professional integrity is under scrutiny, and they should respond to this.

Advise the candidates that the standardised patient should be giving them ongoing feedback throughout the consultation. For example, if they are explaining a procedure and the standardised patient is looking puzzled, they are indicating to the candidate that the explanation is not clear enough.

If the candidates sense a mismatch between the patient's words and their behaviour or appearance, they will often find it very useful to comment on this. If they are accurate in their observations, the standardised patient is likely to reward them with some further verbal explanation. This may give them crucial information to help them to manage the situation more effectively.

> *Candidate:* 'You say everything is going fine at home, but . . . well, to be honest, you look really sad right now . . .'
> *Standardised patient:* '. . . do I? Well, I suppose it's all just a bit difficult at the moment . . .'
> *Candidate:* 'Difficult?'
> *Standardised patient:* '. . . Well, yeah . . . my husband . . . well, since he lost his job . . . you know, he's just been . . . sort of . . . well, I don't know . . . irritable.'

In this way, the candidate has a whole area to explore with the patient that should always be relevant as the standardised patients are trained to respond appropriately to such interventions.

No candidate should lose marks on the introduction. There are often marks given for an appropriate introduction, including for some or all of the following:

> giving their name and role
> checking the name and date of birth of the patient
> indicating the purpose of the interaction
> gaining consent for the consultation
> referring to confidentiality appropriately.

This should be a very straightforward part of the consultation, and in some ways the only part that candidates can actually practise. In some more advanced assessments, they may find that they are not able to give their practised introduction, but if they have the basic principles firmly in their mind, they should be able to give enough of an introduction as is appropriate.

Encourage them to try to relax and approach the standardised patient much as they would approach an actual patient. The examination or interview task is unlikely to be significantly different to a task that they could face in their work or future work situation. However, they must also remember that they are in an assessment situation, which means that while they are carrying out a normal consultation they need to be continually gauging what information they need to make overt to the examiner that they perhaps would not make overt to a patient in an actual consultation. For example, a standardised patient may present with a problem for which the management options are extensive. In reality, if they would not be able to cover all the information in a single consultation, they would simply make another appointment. Good practice may or may not suggest that they would tell the patient exactly what they were intending to deal with in the following appointment. In the assessment situation, however, they definitely need to indicate to the patient what their plan of action is. This is so that the examiner is informed about their management plan.

They may also use this technique if they find that they are running out of time in their consultation. For example, if they realise they will not have time to complete their tasks, advise them to explain this to the simulated patient,

*Candidate:* 'We are running out of time but I still have several things I would like to explore with you. Could we make another appointment so that we can discuss some more about how you are feeling about work, and also maybe have a look at some lifestyle changes that may help to bring your blood pressure down ... you know, things like your diet and, of course ... your smoking! We have many ways we can help you cut down your smoking ... can we discuss that next week maybe?'

In this way, although they have failed to cover these aspects in the consultation, the examiner at least knows that they are considering the impact of work, diet and smoking on the patient's blood pressure.

Finally, remind them that if they feel that a station involving a standardised patient has not gone as well as they had hoped, they should try to clear the experience from their mind before moving on to the next station. It is often more difficult to do this, as a personal interaction usually touches more deeply than a written assessment. However, it is also worth telling the candidates that it is often very difficult for them to gauge how well they have performed at these stations, as, for example, the standardised patient may have been instructed to behave in a certain way no matter what strategies the candidates may employ. The examiner will be marking the candidate's responses and attempts at strategies, not specifically how successful they were with the patient. Equally a candidate may feel that they had built up a great rapport with the patient, but in fact may have misread the question and omitted, for example, to tell them the treatment options available. This part of the question might have carried a significant amount of the available marks and so, by leaving it out, the candidate may fail the station. Therefore, it is essential that, instead of trying to evaluate the last station, candidates move on and approach the next one with fresh eyes.

### Reflection on assessment situations

In essence, the use of simulated patients to assess candidates is less predictable than using a multiple-choice questionnaire, for example. Because of this, it is important that you allow, if possible, some opportunity for the candidates to reflect on their own performance. Human interaction offers up so many variables that it is impossible to obtain completely objective responses from either the candidates or the examiners.

If a candidate is able to analyse their own strengths and weaknesses within a consultation, they are demonstrating the potential to learn from their own experiences and those of others. If they show no insight into their own capabilities, they will probably be less likely to develop their full potential. This additional information about a candidate may or may not be taken into account when awarding the final grade or making the recruitment decision.

The decision as to whether to allow some reflective element in the assessment process may not be a decision you are able to make, but if you do have any influence in this, it is a very informative addition to proceedings.

# CHAPTER 14

# Other simulated patient challenges and new developments

*The great thing in the world is not so much where we stand, as in what direction we are moving.*

Oliver Wendell Holmes (1809–1894)

As previously stated, the use of simulated patients in healthcare training and assessment is limited only by the imagination, and it is impossible, in this book, to cover all ways in which they are currently used, let alone all of the potential uses.

## THE BLURRY BOUNDARIES BETWEEN REAL AND SIMULATED

It can be assumed that we all are patients or users of healthcare provision at some point in our lives. However, some people are obliged to have more interaction with health and social care than others. The experience of these people is invaluable in teaching our healthcare professionals about dealing with their clients. However, additional challenges can be presented when using actual patients as simulated patients.

Actual patients or people with additional functional challenges are invaluable for sharing their experiences of actual disability, illness, treatment and of communication within health and social care settings. However, the work of the simulated patient is different, and while the experience of actual patients or service users can bring so much depth and authenticity to the work, it can also bring with it its own challenges.

### Emotional challenges

Sometimes, patients who have had a difficult pathway through their illness or disability may find that this affects their view of healthcare professionals. It is very important, if a person wishes to work as a simulated patient, whatever their background, that they are able to leave any prejudices, however justified they may be in their own personal lives, outside the classroom or the examination situation. This may be achieved by a one-off conversation or, more effectively, through a series of workshops to explore their own personal journeys and to identify and try to understand any issues that may remain and which cloud their objectivity.

People who have had difficulties coping with mental health issues may make excellent simulated patients as they may have insight into problems that others can only imagine. However, as with a patient with any physical problems, it is important when performing the work that they are well enough to cope with the role of simulated patient.

### Physical/sensory challenges

It is invaluable to use the real experiences of real patients who have been trained to work as simulated patients, particularly those with a sensory impairment. There may be certain additional challenges with this, however, that should be considered before embarking on such work.

Working with a deaf simulated patient can bring great insights into some of the attitudes and challenges they experience within their life. However, much as with a bilingual session, some of the difficulties present with giving feedback. With a bilingual simulator, they are able to give their feedback in English. With a deaf simulator, they continue to use their interpreter to communicate in the feedback session. While this is not a major problem, it is important to think about some of the implications of this, to be better prepared for the session.

If you are using a simulated patient with an evident disability, you should decide whether or not it is better to refer to the disability and incorporate it into the role, or whether it is incidental to the role.

### The challenges of learning disability

It is great experience for practitioners to practise consulting with simulated patients with learning disabilities. The simulators can be recruited from the many theatre and drama groups in this country that are organised specifically for actors with learning disabilities. In this way, the simulated patients will already have some experience of developing and performing a role. The difficulty, once more, can come in the giving of feedback. The concept of giving constructive feedback can be quite alien for some people, and they can often be quite reluctant to appear critical of a practitioner. Once the importance of this is understood, however, their feedback can be very insightful and it can be invaluable for health practitioners.

### The undercover simulated patient

One additional way simulators are currently used may be described as the 'mystery shopper' approach to healthcare education and assessment. Here a simulated patient takes the part of a patient/relative/carer and has an interaction with a healthcare professional who is under the illusion that this is a genuine patient/relative/carer. They may also take the part of a healthcare professional, although this is more difficult to orchestrate.

Simulated patients are currently used in this way in the training of pharmacists who work in retail outlets, as well as in some GP surgeries. They approach the relevant staff members and present a realistic scenario that is dealt with by the healthcare professional. They may then reveal their identity and give the relevant feedback, or they report back to the training provider or assessor, who uses their feedback as part of the practitioner's ongoing professional development training or assessment.

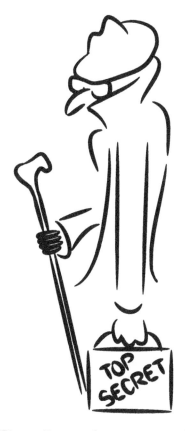

**'Pleez gif to me de aspeereen . . .'**

## AND FINALLY . . .

I hope you have realised the immense potential of using simulated patients within healthcare training. I have only touched on some of the more recent developments; however, I hope it has shown how there really are few limits, apart from those imposed by our resources or ourselves.

I hope you have gained some ideas of different ways to manage both teaching and assessment sessions, to help keep your consultation skills training alive and kicking (with simulated kicks, obviously!).

I hope you have been reassured by learning techniques to manage the potentially difficult situations that inevitably arise when using such an interactive medium.

I hope, above all, that you continue to explore and develop this vibrant and creative way of working and have fun with it! It is there to be played with! Enjoy!

# Consultation skills advanced jargon buster

Here are some of the more common terms you may hear used in the field of consultation skills training. Some of them are probably very familiar to you; if so, please don't feel patronised!

**Acronyms** – healthcare practitioners are taught many acronyms to help them structure their questioning within a consultation. The most common of these can be found in Chapter 5.

**Active listening** – this describes the ways in which the practitioner shows the patient that they are really listening to them (e.g. nodding, head tilting, facial expression and verbal acknowledgements such as 'mm . . . right . . .').

**Acute** – in healthcare terms, a condition or illness that is short-lived and severe. An acute healthcare setting is a place where short-term conditions are treated.

**Aims/objectives/learning outcomes** – these are often seen as interchangeable, but they each have a slightly different emphasis. An aim is a general statement of intent; it describes the direction in which the session is intended to go in terms of what opportunities it will present. An objective is a more specific statement about how the aims will be reached and what the practitioners should be able to achieve at the end of the session. Learning outcomes are similar to objectives; they are a statement of what it is hoped the practitioners should know, understand and be able to do by the end of the session.

**Body language** – non-verbal behaviour.

**Chronic** – in healthcare terms, a long illness with no reference to the severity of the condition.

**Chunking and checking** – a technique to make sure the patient understands any information they are given. It involves giving the information in small sections and then ascertaining whether or not the patient has understood.

**Circuit** – a series of questions that should be answered in an examination such as an objective structured clinical examination.

**Confidentiality** – it is often important for the practitioner to make the patient aware of the level of confidentiality that is guaranteed within any given interaction. This should be done honestly and clearly.

**Consent/informed consent** – it is essential for practitioners to make sure that a patient agrees to a particular procedure or treatment. In order to agree, they must know and understand exactly what it is that they are agreeing to. It can also be used in a consultation to make sure that the patient agrees to talk with the practitioner, or agrees to being asked certain questions.

**Constructive feedback** – things that could be tried differently are identified and explored for future reference.

**Core competencies** – the basic skills and attitudes essential for a practitioner to demonstrate in order to prove their ability to practise.

**Differential diagnoses/differentials** – the different diagnoses that a practitioner might consider, based on a patient's symptoms and investigations. Gradually each one would be eliminated as more information was gathered, until a final diagnosis is reached.

**Drug history** – the medications taken by a patient, which can include prescribed medication, over-the-counter remedies and illicit drugs.

**Empathy** – the practitioner's ability to genuinely try to understand the world from the patient's point of view. They will demonstrate empathy through a selection of communication skills, both verbal and non-verbal.

**Family history** – an account of any illnesses or conditions that have been suffered by the patient's family.

**History of presenting complaint/problem** – the symptoms and events that have brought the patient to the consultation at this time.

**Management planning** – the part of the consultation where the practitioner (in negotiation with the patient!) decides on a plan of action to deal with the particular problems encountered by the patient.

**Mannequins, high fidelity** – high-fidelity mannequins are life-size models, usually of entire human bodies, that reproduce many bodily functions and movements and are able to respond to certain treatments and interventions in real time.

**Mannequins, low fidelity** – low-fidelity mannequins are life-size models of entire human bodies or body parts that are used in the healthcare professions for the training and assessment of various clinical examination procedures.

**Medical history** – an account of any illnesses or operations the patient has had in the past.

**Mirroring** – a technique whereby a practitioner subtly mimics the body language of the patient in order to help build rapport with the patient.

**Ongoing feedback** – the reactions of the simulated patient that can give information to the practitioner about their own performance.

**Positive feedback** – where the things that the practitioner did well in the session are pointed out to them.

**Practitioner-directed sessions** – also known as masterclasses and improvised sessions, these sessions allow the practitioners to bring along communication difficulties they have experienced or witnessed in practice. A scenario is developed from these difficulties and the group have the chance to explore strategies to deal with the challenges.

**Primary care** – includes any healthcare providers who provide a first point of call for a patient (e.g. general practitioners, dentists, pharmacists, walk-in centres).

**Questioning styles: closed question** – a question that can be answered with a one-word (usually yes or no) or very brief answer. Closed questions are used when specific and detailed clinical information is needed. For example:

'Is the pain keeping you awake at night?'

**Questioning styles: leading question** – a question that guides the person to answer in a certain way. This is only useful when the information has already been gained, as a kind of summary. For example:

'So you want some stronger painkillers?'

**Questioning styles: multiple questions** – when a practitioner asks one question and then asks another before the patient has had a chance to answer the first question. For example:

'So how long have you had the pain? Has it got worse since you first got it?'

**Questioning styles: open question** – a question that cannot be answered with a one-word or very brief answer but invites a more expansive response instead. These are used effectively when gathering information from the patient. For example:

'Can you tell me a bit more about the pain.'

**Safety-netting** – where the practitioner makes sure they have made follow-up arrangements if necessary and/or they have given the patient guidance as to what to do should the patient require further help with their particular problem.

**Secondary care** – the healthcare providers who treat patients after they have been referred by primary care practitioners. They are based in hospitals or in the community.

**Signposting** – a technique whereby the practitioner indicates to the patient what they would like to talk about next and links different areas of questioning. For example:

'I would like to ask you a few questions now about your lifestyle.'

**Station** – this is one question in an examination such as an objective structured clinical examination.

**Summarising, long summaries** – the practitioner summarises what has been discussed in the consultation and what they have understood about the information they have heard. Long summaries have many functions in the context of the medical consultation, including (1) they show the patient that they have been listened to; (2) they give the opportunity for the patient to correct or add to the information; and (3) they can help the practitioner make sense of the information

**Summarising, short summaries/reflection/paraphrasing** – the practitioner echoes the patient's own words in an attempt to encourage them to elaborate further. This is effective if some silence is left afterwards for the patient to continue. For example:

*Simulated patient:*   'It's really beginning to get me down . . .'
*Practitioner:*   'Get you down?'
*Simulated patient:*   'Yes . . . I mean, I get so tired . . . and then I get irritable with the kids . . .'

This also makes it clear to the patient that the practitioner is listening. Summarising in this way can also be used to link parts of the consultation together and to create signposts. For example:

'You said your mother had told you to take the antacids . . . can I ask you a bit about her health and that of the rest of your family? Has your mother ever suffered from chest pains?'

# Sample scenario briefs

## SAMPLE BRIEF 1: BASIC CONSULTATION SKILLS TRAINING – HISTORY TAKING

This is a scenario that could be used for early consultation skills training sessions. Basic skills such as introductions, summaries and the use of open and closed questions can be practised. The session can be kept at this level, but if appropriate it can also be used to look at more sophisticated skills, such as showing empathy and making links between psychological factors and physical symptoms. The scenario can be varied in many ways to increase or decrease challenge.

### Potential learning points

- ➤ **Medical** – exploring differential diagnoses around headaches
- ➤ **Psychological** – exploring the psychological impact of physical symptoms and exploring the possible psychological basis of physical symptoms
- ➤ **Social** – appreciating the impact on the individual of complex social pressures
- ➤ **Communication** – practising the consultation skills needed to take a holistic history and exploring the techniques and value of demonstrating empathy to a patient
- ➤ **Teamwork** – exploring other support mechanisms available in the community
- ➤ **Ethical** – confidentiality
- ➤ **Health promotion** – discussing appropriateness of ad hoc health promotion around smoking
- ➤ **Professional integrity** – less relevant

### Simulated patient's brief

- ➤ Name: any
- ➤ Age range: your own age
- ➤ Gender: any
- ➤ Ethnicity: any

### Setting of interaction
This consultation takes place in the general practitioner surgery.

### Reason for interaction
You have come to see the doctor because you have been getting headaches for some time, and you are beginning to worry about the cause.

### Background
You are normally fit and well, but for the last 6 months you have been getting painful headaches that have been increasing both in frequency and in severity. The headaches are usually across the top of your head, and it feels as though a great weight is pressing down on them. Occasionally you also experience sharp pains behind your eyes. You are not sure exactly when you started to notice them as a problem, as you think they started about 6 months ago, maybe once a week, and have gradually become more frequent. You have not noticed any other symptoms that you think could be directly related to the headaches, although you are feeling quite tired for much of the time. There does not seem to be a pattern to the headaches. They can occur at any time of day, although you think they are often worse in the evening. They have never woken you up at night.

You have been taking over-the-counter medication, such as paracetamol. This used to relieve the symptoms, but for the last 2 months they have merely taken the edge off the pain, but not eased it completely.

When you get a headache, you carry on doing what you are doing, because you have to, but you wish you could just lie down to ease the pain. On a scale of 1–10, the pain around the top of your head is about a 4. The pains that you get occasionally behind your eyes is about an 8. You have no nausea and have not vomited. The headaches are not disturbing your sleep. Your appetite is unchanged. You have no visual disturbances.

### Social history
You are married with three children (their ages appropriate to your own age). Your partner was made redundant a year ago when the local plastics factory went into liquidation. S/he has been unable to find work since then. S/he is becoming increasingly frustrated, and your relationship is quite tense at times because of this.

You work day shifts as a packer at a warehouse. You have worked there for the last 9 years. The company is about to be taken over by a large American corporation, and there are rumours of inevitable redundancies. You are very worried about this as you are barely managing to pay the bills on one wage, let alone if you lost your job too.

Your parents live nearby and are becoming more and more dependent on you for their shopping and housework, although they still manage their own personal care and cooking. They never accepted your partner, and so you shoulder the bulk of the responsibility for this.

### *Lifestyle*

You smoke 20 cigarettes per day and have done since your late teens. You used to enjoy going out with friends for a drink but have not enough money to do this very often now. Also your partner rarely wants to go out since losing their job. You do not take any formal exercise, but feel that you never stop running around after people, so you don't really need to. You have a 'normal' diet. A typical day would be coffee for breakfast, coffee and cake in the morning break. You usually get a sandwich in the canteen at lunchtime, then have a meat, two-veg dinner most nights, which your partner cooks. You also eat a lot of snacks, including crisps and chocolate.

### *Past medical history*

You had your appendix out when you were aged 15. You have no other significant illnesses or operations.

### *Family history*

Both your parents suffer increasingly with osteoarthritis, which has significantly disabled them in recent years.

### *Medication*

Paracetamol when required.

### *Allergies*

You have no known allergies.

### *Temperament*

You are usually a positive person, not afraid of hard work, and you are always trying to find the silver lining in every cloud. However, over the last year you have found yourself increasingly worn down by the pressures you have been under through your partner's redundancy and resulting state of mind, your parents' ill health, your own work and the general day-to-day demands of caring for your children and managing the home.

### *Ideas*

You don't really have any ideas what is causing these headaches.

You have never been the sort of person who dwells on things like this, very much believing that the best policy is to ignore things and they should go away.

### *Concerns*

You are vaguely anxious about what is causing the headaches, but you are more concerned about what would happen if they continued to get worse, and you weren't able to do all you do for everyone.

### Expectations

You rarely come to the doctor's and you assume that they will be able to tell you what is wrong and give you some treatment, probably tablets, to make the headaches better. If further investigation is suggested, you may become anxious as you have such a lot on; you just want a 'quick fix'.

### Behaviour

You are an amiable person, although clearly stressed by the demands of your life. You should remain pleasant and cooperative throughout the consultation and should answer questions in a friendly and open manner (although not giving too much information at a time). You should appear worn down by life's demands but still wanting to fulfil your responsibilities. You are keen to put a stop to the headaches, and would seem even more stressed by any suggestion of further investigation.

### Impact on life

You are still doing your daily activities, but everything is much more effort because of the headaches.

### Feelings

You are feeling rundown and anxious most of the time.

### Variations

None.

### Timeline

➤ 6 months ago: headaches started
➤ 2 months ago: painkillers no longer adequate.

### Opening statement

'I've been getting these awful headaches … they're really beginning to get me down.'

### Practitioner's brief

You are a student attached to the general practitioner surgery. You have been asked to take a history from a patient. S/he is an infrequent attender and has not been seen for about 4 years, which was when s/he had a bout of flu.

### SAMPLE BRIEF 2: DIFFUSING A POTENTIALLY ANGRY SITUATION

This is a scenario that could be used in a more advanced communication skills session, focusing on dealing with a distressed relative, and diffusing a potentially angry situation.

The scenario can be varied in many ways to increase or decrease challenge.

**Potential learning points**

➤ **Medical** – less relevant but potential for exploring effects of lack of adequate care on patient
➤ **Psychological** – to appreciate the underlying feelings that drive behaviour and to understand the importance of acknowledging these feelings empathically
➤ **Social** – to appreciate the effects of the social support/isolation a patient may have
➤ **Communication** – to explore different ways to effectively diffuse potentially angry situations and to practise breaking bad news
➤ **Teamwork** – to explore the importance of good teamwork in patient care
➤ **Ethical** – to address the issue of patient confidentiality, while remaining empathic towards a relative
➤ **Health promotion** – less relevant
➤ **Professional integrity** – to explore ways of maintaining professional integrity when under the pressure of complaints about a colleague.

**Simulated patient's brief**

➤ Name: any
➤ Age range: 40–70 years
➤ Gender: any
➤ Ethnicity: any

*Setting of interaction*

This consultation takes place on the elderly admissions ward of your local hospital where your mother, Mrs Ella MacDiarmid, is currently an inpatient.

*Reason for interaction*

You had come to visit your mother, who was admitted 3 weeks ago following a fall at home. You were told yesterday that she would be discharged today. Your mother has had a very miserable time here, and now you have arrived to take her home, only to find that her discharge papers have not been prepared and her medications are not ready. Your mother takes a number of different medications, which she was told to bring in with her when she was first admitted to hospital. This means that she no longer has any medication, either at home or in her possession in the hospital, as the nurses dispense medication from a central source during patients' time in hospital.

Yesterday a nurse told you to come after 4 p.m. because that would give them time for the consultant to see your mother, for the discharge arrangements to be made, for the necessary paperwork to be prepared and for your mother's medication to be collected from pharmacy. You decided to use your last day without your mother to visit a housebound friend in town and have only just arrived, at 5 p.m.

### Background

Your mother had lived alone since the death of your father 11 years ago. She has become increasingly disabled with chronic airways disease, arthritis and early Parkinson's disease. She has been unable to manage at home for a while and you had a few months where you were continually calling round to check up on her and help her with her chores. Eventually, you decided a year ago to give up work and go to live with your mother. You have let out your own house to provide a small income, but are now reliant on benefits and your small savings to survive.

You do not want your mother to go into residential accommodation, but you are, if you are honest with yourself, struggling with the whole situation, as you are having to give her a lot of care, and you rarely get a break. Three weeks ago, while you were in the bath, your mother fell. You were mortified and felt very guilty about the accident. She was very distressed, and was admitted to hospital. No bones were broken, although she was badly bruised and very shaken. Soon after arriving in the hospital, she contracted a chest infection and has been quite poorly.

### Social history

You were divorced 16 years ago and never married again. You have no children. You used to work as a librarian, which you enjoyed doing, but you gave this up to care for your mother.

### Lifestyle

You don't smoke and you never have. You seldom drink. You have a healthy diet, with plenty of fresh fruit and vegetables. You were training for the Great North Run but now, as you have to get a sitter every time you need to leave your mother, you can only do this for the necessities, such as shopping trips.

### Temperament

You are usually quite calm and reasonable, only very occasionally, under extreme provocation, losing your temper. When you lose your temper you tend to become less articulate and you express your feelings in frustrated rather than raging terms.

### Ideas

You feel very guilty about your mother's accident, but you also blame the hospital for the length of stay she has had on the ward. You noticed a visitor to the patient in a neighbouring bed who was coughing and sneezing during their visit. You think this is probably how your mother contracted the chest infection.

You feel that you have given up your job to make sure that your mother is properly cared for, and that you have entrusted her to the care of the hospital, only to find that the care she has received is, in your opinion, very poor.

### Concerns

You have a number of concerns about your mother's stay on the ward:

➤ Your mother has spent 2 out of the 3 weeks in a mixed bay, and finds the situation extremely embarrassing.

➤ Your mother has complained that the staff often seem impatient with her when she needs to go to the toilet, and it seems to be pot luck whether there is anyone to help her eat her lunch. She often has bread with no butter because she can't open the plastic butter container, and she leaves food because she struggles to use the cutlery.

➤ Twice when you have visited your mother, you found her ravenously hungry. She had then explained that on one occasion, her meal had been left at the end of the bed and she had been unable to reach it. On another occasion, she had been asleep while dinner had been brought and cleared away, and was not offered anything else to eat.

➤ You had witnessed a nurse picking up a bottle from the bed of the man in the corner, splashing urine on the bed table. She wiped it with a tissue, and then placed his lunch on it.

➤ Your mother has been very unhappy on the ward, and is absolutely desperate to come home. You have tried to pacify her by promising that she would be coming home today. You haven't wanted to complain to anyone before as you felt that your mother is in a vulnerable position and you would fear leaving her alone on the ward, if you had complained.

### Expectations

You are expecting the practitioner to organise everything to enable you to take your mother home.

### Behaviour

You have no intention of complaining about anything when you arrive on the ward, thinking that you just want to get your mother home as soon as possible. When the practitioner explains that it will not be possible for you to take your mother home today, you become very upset and angry about the fact and your anger escalates into you complaining about everything that has happened to your mother.

If the practitioner seems defensive or disinterested in your concerns, you will become more and more angry, maybe even deciding to make an official complaint.

If the practitioner seems apologetic and empathic, you will continue to be upset, but this will be more likely to be a distressed upset rather than an angry one.

If the practitioner is very empathic, you may even feel you can share some of your feelings of guilt and your struggles in managing to look after your mother.

*Timeline*

➤ 11 years ago: your mother was widowed.
➤ 1 year ago: you moved in to care for her.
➤ 3 weeks ago: your mother had a fall and was admitted to hospital.

*Opening statement*

> 'I don't want to complain, but . . . oh, I don't know . . . this is just the last straw!'

### Practitioner's brief

You are a staff nurse working on the elderly admissions ward of the local hospital, where a 75-year-old lady, Mrs Ella MacDiarmid, was admitted 3 weeks ago, following a fall at home. While on the ward she contracted a chest infection, and has been quite poorly. She is much improved now and very keen to go home.

You have just come back to work after 3 days off. You have just been told that, although she is well enough to go home, in fact the doctor had not signed the paperwork in time and the order for her medication was not sent to pharmacy in time. Pharmacy is now closed.

You see the lady sitting by her bed, dressed ready to go, as her son/daughter arrives on the ward. There is no possibility of her going home today as there is no way you can get her medication sorted out. You approach her son/daughter to explain the situation.

### SAMPLE BRIEF 3: BILINGUAL CONSULTATION WITH FAMILY MEMBER AS INTERPRETER

This is a scenario that can be used for the more advanced consultation skills around managing a third-party bilingual consultation. The session can be used to look at many different issues arising when a patient does not speak English. The scenario can be varied in many ways to increase or decrease challenge.

### Potential learning points

➤ **Medical** – reaching a diagnosis or formulating a management plan when information gathering is difficult
➤ **Psychological** – exploring the presenting family dynamics and how they can affect a consultation; identifying power relationships and the vulnerability some people experience as a result of their limited understanding of English and the organisation of English society; appreciating the cultural implications of having, and discussing, certain symptoms
➤ **Social** – realising the social isolation a lack of understanding of English can produce
➤ **Communication** – logistics of communicating in a third-party

consultation; issues around communicating with someone who does not speak or understand English
➤ **Team-working** – looking at access to interpreting services, exploring the importance of building the relationship with the interpreter
➤ **Ethical** – many ethical issues, including confidentiality and obtaining informed consent
➤ **Professional integrity** – exploring issues of professionalism inherent in working with various interpreters within the consultation

## Simulated patient's brief
➤ Name: any
➤ Age range: your own age
➤ Gender: any
➤ Ethnicity: any, but please make adjustments to the role according to cultural differences

### Setting of interaction
This interaction can take place in a general practitioner, nurse practitioner, health centre or A&E setting.

### Reason for interaction
You have noticed some bright-red blood on the toilet paper, immediately after passing stools.

### Background
You first noticed this about 2 weeks ago. You were very worried, but you were too embarrassed to do anything about it. Since then it has happened four times and so, finally, you have decided that you must find out what is causing it.

You have never noticed any blood in the toilet bowl or in your stools, but only on the toilet paper. It is only a very small amount of bright red blood. Your anus is slightly painful, especially on passing stools. You have no constipation or diarrhoea. You have never had anything like this before.

### Social history
You arrived in Britain 4 weeks ago to begin a 3-month visit to your cousin, who is a postgraduate student here. Your cousin is finishing their PhD and intends to return to your homeland on completion. Your parents encouraged you to take advantage of the fact that your cousin is here, in order to have a cheap trip to England. They had hoped that you would learn some English while you were here, but you have made friends within your cousin's social circle, which consists mainly of people from your own country. You have never been close to your cousin, and in fact you have little in common with each other. Your cousin is very studious, conscientious and serious. You are more gregarious and you want to go out and experience English nightlife.

### Lifestyle

You have enjoyed experiencing what you see very much as English culture in the form of fast food. You smoke 10 cigarettes per day. You have developed a liking for English beer, and drink a couple of pints three or four times a week. You have borrowed a bicycle to get around the city and are reasonably fit.

### Past medical history

You have no significant past medical history.

### Family history

You have no significant family history.

### Medication

You do not take any medication.

### Allergies

You have no allergies.

### Temperament

You are normally a fairly outgoing sort of person. This is a little tempered at the moment by the relationship you have with your cousin. You feel that your cousin resents you being there, but has no choice as they have been ordered to accommodate you by his/her parents.

You are also subdued by the fact that you are very worried about the cause of the bleeding. You have not told your cousin about the reason for your need to see a health professional, as you feel that your cousin would be very judgemental of you. You had even considered coming alone and trying to manage by yourself but you realised that you need your cousin to interpret for you.

It is very difficult to talk about such intimate things with your cousin, who gets easily embarrassed and flustered by such subjects.

### Ideas

You do not know what could have caused this bleeding. You have recently had several sexual encounters and think it may be as a result of these.

### Concerns

You are worried that the bleeding may be an indication of something serious. You have a friend whose mother died of bowel cancer last year and you are scared your symptoms are due to this, even though you don't know what her symptoms were.

### Expectations

You are hoping for some reassurance from the practitioner. You assume they will need to do some investigations to discover the cause of the symptoms.

### *Behaviour*

You should appear not to understand much of what the health practitioner says, relying solely on the interpretations of your cousin. You should be quite open and descriptive about your symptoms, albeit in your native language.

### *Impact on life*

You are still doing your normal activities.

### *Feelings*

You feel a little anxious.

### *Timeline*

➤ 4 weeks ago: you came to Britain.
➤ 2 weeks ago: you first noticed the blood.

### Simulated relative's brief

➤ Name: any
➤ Age range: your own age
➤ Gender: any
➤ Ethnicity: any, but please make adjustments to the role according to cultural differences

### *Setting of interaction*

This interaction can take place in a general practitioner, nurse practitioner, health centre or A&E setting.

### *Reason for interaction*

You have come to act as interpreter for your cousin who has come to stay with you for 3 months. They have only been in Britain for 4 weeks and have learnt almost no English.

### *Background*

Your cousin has told you they need to see a healthcare practitioner and has told you that you must come to interpret for them. Your cousin would not tell you what the problem was when you asked.

### *Social history*

Your parents insisted that you should act as host to your cousin, who wanted to come to Britain for a few months. You protested, as you have a lot of work to do for your postgraduate course, but they insisted that you should do it for the sake of family relations.

You are not close to your cousin; in fact, you have little in common with each other. You are very studious and serious. Your cousin is more gregarious and wants to go out and experience English nightlife. You are not very assertive and often find you have to accommodate your cousin's whims at the expense of your own work and life.

### Lifestyle

You eat a healthy diet. You do not smoke. You do not drink alcohol. You are fit, cycling everywhere and swimming three times a week.

### Temperament

You are a very shy, unassuming person. You have one close friend, but generally you find it quite hard to talk to people you don't know. You are very polite and respectful of people generally. You prefer your own company to noisy, busy environments. You feel very resentful of your cousin's presence. This is made worse by the fact that you are a little intimidated by them. You find yourself giving in to their demands continually. You have no respect for your cousin, thinking them superficial and brash.

### Behaviour

You have no idea of what you will be required to interpret. You should appear very uncomfortable discussing your cousin's symptoms, both with your cousin and also when required to interpret them for the healthcare practitioner.

You should be quite reluctant to interpret some of the things your cousin says. You should use euphemisms whenever possible and talk around the subjects without getting to the point where appropriate. You are excruciatingly embarrassed by the whole situation.

### Opening statement

'I'm just here to translate for my cousin . . . s/he doesn't speak any English.'

### Practitioner's brief

You are about to see a patient who has just registered as a temporary resident. You have no other information about them.

### SAMPLE BRIEF 4: IMPROVISED FORUM SESSION EXPLORING SENSITIVE COMMUNICATION BETWEEN ANCILLARY STAFF AND PATIENTS

This is a situation that can be presented in a forum session to illustrate the difficulties that can arise from well-meaning comments in a highly emotionally charged situation. It is intended to help practitioners explore ways of recognising and dealing with distress in patients.

This is intended to be an improvised forum presentation, so there is no script as such, but the two simulated patients are expected to interact with each other according to the guidelines in their briefs.

The facilitator should stop the interaction after a few minutes, when the insensitivity of the domestic and the frustration of the patient have been clearly expressed. The session can then proceed either by a full-group hot-seating and directing exercise or by sending the two simulated patients to separate groups.

### Character brief for forum session

This is an unscripted forum session. Based on the following background information and suggested phrases, please begin an interaction with the member of staff until the facilitator asks you to stop.

You will then be asked to stay in role and take direction from the group as indicated by the facilitator. On the facilitator's instructions, you will then be asked to resume the interaction with the member of staff according to the advice you will have been given. This process may be repeated.

➤ Name: James MacIntyre
➤ Age range: 30–50 years
➤ Gender: male
➤ Ethnicity: any (but please change name to culturally appropriate one if necessary)

### Setting of interaction

This conversation takes place in a single room in the hospice where you are a patient.

### Reason for interaction

You are lying in bed, reading. The domestic has come into the room to clean it.

### Background

You are a new patient in the hospice. You have been diagnosed with terminal lung cancer but you do not know how long you have left to live.

### Social history

You have been married for 4 years; you have a 2-year-old son and your wife is pregnant with your second child.

You have recently had to give up your job as a salesman. You had only been in this job for a few months, so you have little entitlement to sick pay. You have no life insurance policy. Your main anxiety at the moment is your family.

### Lifestyle

You lived quite a 'wild' life before you met your wife and had a family. You used to smoke and drink heavily but gave up smoking with her encouragement. Your drinking was also greatly reduced, although you did still go out with your mates once a week, when you would drink about 8 pints or more. You used to use recreational drugs, like cannabis, cocaine, speed and Ecstasy before you met her, but have only smoked cannabis a couple of times since.

### Past medical history
You always seemed fit and well until now.

### Family history
You have no family history of any major illnesses.

### James's perspective
### Temperament
You are a melancholic, taciturn person. You have never been the sort of person who can readily talk about their feelings. However, you are feeling rather vulnerable at the moment, having just come into the hospice a few days ago. It is almost as though you have suddenly taken in the enormity of the situation and this has left you quite unguarded and open to conversation.

### Ideas
You are feeling guilty about letting your wife and children down, having for the first time in your life felt committed to a relationship. You are regretting the wild life you lived before you met your wife and the way you used to abuse your health and body. You suddenly feel that you have caused your illness and feel that through this you are destroying not only your own life but also the lives of the family you love.

### Concerns
You are terrified of dying, but at the moment the biggest worry that you have is leaving your family and how they will cope without you.

### Expectations
You weren't expecting any visitors today, as your wife has had to go to see her mother, who is also unwell. You were feeling miserable and lonely, and so when the domestic, whose name you don't even know, came in, you were quite relieved to be able to talk, albeit in a morose manner.

### Behaviour
You are normally taciturn, but will respond with unusual candour to the questions of the domestic. You will not expand on your answers very much, but you will be surprisingly open and honest. She will use the things you say to prompt her own musings about her own situation. You are so engrossed in your own guilt and grief that you will just politely nod and acknowledge the chatterings of the domestic, maybe occasionally asking a question out of politeness.

Please begin the conversation more or less as follows:

*Domestic* 'Now then, how are you today?'
*Patient* 'Bit fed up, I suppose.'
*Domestic* 'Aah . . . what's the matter, love?'

*Patient*  'Oh, I don't know ... just keep thinking about the missus and that, you know ... feeling guilty and that ...'

*Domestic*  'Oh, you don't want to be feeling guilty, love ... we could all beat ourselves up feeling guilty for what we've done and haven't done ... doesn't do anyone any good does it ...'

Please try to include some of the following phrases in your conversation with the domestic. These do not have to be learnt, they are only to give you a general feel for the gist of the conversation:

'I guess you could say this is not my finest hour!'

'I'm just not having a great day ...'

'How the hell is she going to cope?'

'It's all my fault ...'

'You think you're so bloody invincible when you're young, don't you ... all the stuff I did and now look what it's led to ...'

'How will she manage?'

'Just when you get something worth living for, this has to happen ...'

'How can I have been so stupid?'

You will answer questions and appear politely interested in what the domestic is talking about, but you are preoccupied with your own situation. Really you wish she would go away and leave you alone, but you would never say such a thing.

### Character brief for forum session: Marion Clarke

This is an unscripted forum session. Based on the following background information and suggested phrases, please begin an interaction with the patient until the facilitator asks you to stop.

You will then be asked to stay in role and take direction from the group as indicated by the facilitator. On the facilitator's instructions, you will then be asked to resume the interaction with the patient according to the advice you will have been given. This process may be repeated.

➤ Name: Marion Clarke
➤ Age range: 30–60 years
➤ Gender: female
➤ Ethnicity: any (but please change name to culturally appropriate one if necessary)

### *Setting of interaction*

This conversation takes place in a single room in the hospice where you work as a domestic.

### Reason for interaction

You have just gone into one of the single rooms to clean it. You see the patient lying in bed and you begin a conversation with him, as you usually do with the patients as you are cleaning their rooms.

### Social history

You have worked as a domestic at your local hospice for about 9 years. This is only one of your jobs. Since your husband was made redundant 2 years ago, you have had to take on more work to pay the mortgage. You also work in a pub three evenings a week, and you sell cosmetics in your local neighbourhood.

You really enjoy all your work, although you get tired and feel permanently stressed about your home situation. You feel that your husband should try harder to get another job, but you suspect he is suffering from mild depression, as he seems to be becoming less and less motivated to do anything. You have two teenaged boys who need continual nagging to do their schoolwork or give any help around the house. You also visit your own parents daily, as they need more and more help with daily living. Your father has Alzheimer's disease and your mother struggles to cope.

### Lifestyle

You smoke 20 cigarettes a day, and you have been trying to cut down because of the cost as much as anything, but with all the additional stress of your current situation you have not been at all successful.

You do enjoy going to the local social club with your husband a couple of times a week, and you think it is important that people get the chance to 'let their hair down' every once in a while.

### Marion's perspective

#### Temperament

You are a very kind and friendly person, enjoying chatting with the people you meet in the course of your work. You always ask how the patients are feeling when you come into their rooms to clean them, and you will chat to them as you go about your work.

You always try to be positive towards the patients, trying to encourage them to look on the bright side of life.

### Behaviour

You ask the patient a lot of questions, but you merely use his answers as a prompt to talk about your own life. You feel very sorry for the patients' situations, but at this point in your life you are quite absorbed in your own troubles, which you don't mind sharing with the patients if they seem interested. You want to talk about your troubles, but not in a self-pitying way. Rather, you see it as a way to make the patients feel that they are not the only ones having a hard time.

You are a very chatty person, responding to the slightest prompt from the patient with a story, complaint or anecdote from your own life. You are completely oblivious to the fact that you may be making the patient feel worse by your chatter.

Please begin the conversation more or less as follows:

*Domestic*   'Now then, how are you today?'
*Patient*   'Bit fed up, I suppose.'
*Domestic*   'What's the matter, love?'
*Patient*   'Oh I don't know . . . just keep thinking about the missus and that, you know . . . feeling guilty and that . . .'
*Domestic*   'Oh, you don't want to be feeling guilty, love . . . we could all beat ourselves up feeling guilty for what we've done and haven't done . . . doesn't do anyone any good does it . . .'

Please try to include some of the following phrases in your conversation with the patient. These do not have to be learnt, they are only to give you a general feel for the gist of the conversation:

'I'm not surprised, it's a difficult time isn't it. Mind you, it's a difficult time of year as well I suppose, you know with Christmas coming up, it's never easy is it . . .'

'I'm so exhausted, I was round at my mother's last night . . . dad's playing up again . . . losing it a bit . . . so hard for her to cope with him . . . you'll never guess what he did last week . . .'

'You shouldn't be blaming yourself . . .'

'Its easy to blame ourselves for what happens . . . I mean I blame myself for those two lazy lumps of teenagers I've got at home . . . my mother always said I was spoiling them . . . making a rod for my own back . . .'

'Oh, you always think people will never manage but they always do . . . look at my mum . . . dad was always the strong one . . . she never paid a bill, changed a light bulb or anything in her life but she has to do it all now . . . I mean, obviously I help a bit, but it's amazing how she's managing . . .'

'Oh, I know, smoking's a killer isn't it . . . I have been trying to give up for years, but it's easier said than done isn't it . . . you shouldn't be feeling guilty about it . . . it's all very well doctors and the like going on about it . . . when you've got a stressful life it's not as easy as they make out to stop smoking . . . makes me laugh here, you're not allowed to smoke anywhere in the grounds, and you see relatives skulking around in the bushes for a crafty fag . . . well, it's not surprising is it, I mean it's a stressful place isn't it.'

You should chatter away, but not in a completely over-the-top way. You are a kind person, and you are really only trying to make him feel better. You do not realise that you could be making him feel worse by the things you are saying.

### SAMPLE BRIEF 5: MENTAL HEALTH SCENARIO – MULTIPLE USES

This is a scenario that could be used for advanced consultation skills training. Practitioners can practise communicating with a patient who has quite serious mental health problems. The session can be used on many levels, and adapted to explore many different challenges. The scenario can be varied in many ways to increase or decrease challenge.

### Potential learning points

➤ **Medical** – use of appropriate models of therapeutic interventions (e.g. cognitive behavioural therapy)
➤ **Psychological** – exploring issues around living with a serious mental health problem
➤ **Social** – exploring the impact of social support systems around the patient and exploring the impact of the patient's mental health needs on the social network around him
➤ **Communication** – practising the consultation skills needed to take a holistic history and exploring the techniques and value of demonstrating empathy to a patient
➤ **Teamwork** – exploring other support mechanisms available in the community
➤ **Health promotion** – appropriate health promotion interventions
➤ **Ethical** – explore issues of capacity and informed consent
➤ **Professional integrity** – exploring issues of professionalism when working with people with mental health problems.

### Simulated patient's brief

➤ Name: Conor Carlton
➤ Age range: 20–25 years
➤ Gender: male
➤ Ethnicity: any

### Setting of interaction

This conversation takes place in your living room.

### Reason for interaction

You were discharged from an acute unit where you had been for 3 months following a psychotic episode during which you stopped eating.

### Background

You have suffered with schizophrenia since your late teens. This effectively means that you hear voices talking to you when there is no one speaking to you. These voices are inside your head, which you know, but they are very real to you and you often feel the need to act on what they are saying. The voices are of three women – you recognise them individually and they each talk to you about different things.

The voices tend to be derogatory, telling you that you smell, that you are ugly, that no one wants to be with you. They also focus on food, and other substances that are potentially poisonous to you. They imply that 'people' want to see you dead because you are so unpleasant.

At other times your voices tell you that because you smell, you should stay away from people because they won't be able to stand the smell. This results in you avoiding social contact, and generally you lead quite an isolated life.

You hear voices constantly, but with the help of the medication are able to deal with them most of the time. Sometimes the voices become too persistent to ignore. This is what happened this time. Your voices often tell you that food is rancid and you shouldn't eat it. This time you did stop eating for a time, and your mother arranged for you to be admitted into hospital.

### Social history

You live with your parents who both work. They provide general supervision for you. Your brother lives nearby and he is your main social contact. You often go to his house in the evenings to watch TV or occasionally you will go with him to the local pub. You first became ill 2 months before you were due to take your A-levels. You never completed school and you have never had a job.

### Lifestyle

Your mother provides meals for you. They are healthy meals, although it is often difficult for you to eat them because of the nature of the voices you hear, telling you the food is bad and that it will kill you if you eat it.

You do no specific exercise, but you do go for a lot of walks around the city during the day.

You smoke about 20 cigarettes per day. You don't drink alcohol, choosing Coke when you go for a drink with your brother.

### Past medical history

You were diagnosed with schizophrenia following your second psychotic episode in your late teens.

### Family history

You have no history of any psychiatric illnesses in the family.

### Medication
You are on a new antipsychotic drug called olanzapine.

### Allergies
You have no known allergies.

### Temperament
You are a quiet man, made more so by the nature of the voices you hear, which lower your confidence even more. You live a quiet life, spending most of your days either watching TV or going for walks around your neighbourhood. You occasionally get agitated by the voices, but on the whole you accept them, sometimes acting on what they tell you and sometimes not.

### Ideas
You know you have been diagnosed with schizophrenia and what it means. You can talk quite openly about your voices. You don't know why you believe them and act on what they tell you sometimes.

### Concerns
You have no specific concerns really.

### Expectations
You do not really have any expectations of the practitioner.

### Behaviour
You act in a very 'low-key' way throughout. You are quite flat in your mood, not depressed, but a bit monotone. You talk quite openly about your voices, the sorts of things they say and why you do the things you do. You should answer all questions to the best of your ability, but as you are a bit flat, you will not elaborate over much. You should not smile during the consultation, but you will not look angry or miserable. You may occasionally pause as if a little distracted before answering questions, and if asked you should say that you have been listening to them.

### Opening statement
You do not make an opening statement but you respond to the practitioner's questions.

### Practitioner's brief
You have been asked to visit this patient at home, following their recent discharge from the psychiatric inpatients department. The purpose of the visit can be determined by the learning objectives of the session.

## SAMPLE BRIEF 6: FOR USE IN SIMULATED PATIENT TRAINING SESSIONS

Here is your homework! This is the role we will be working with in the workshops during the first training day. Please could you read and think about how you would develop this role, in preparation for this. (Note: this role has been developed specifically for the purposes of simulated patient training, and as such there are areas left for you to develop yourself. In reality, any scenario you receive should give you all relevant information.)

➤ Name: any
➤ Age range: your own
➤ Gender: any
➤ Ethnicity: any

### Setting of interaction

This interaction takes place in the general practitioner surgery.

### Reason for interaction

You have decided to come to the doctor's as you have a cough that has been going on for 3 weeks and is not getting any better, and you are beginning to feel very tired and rundown as a result of not sleeping.

### Background

You had a bad cold 3 weeks ago and have had this cough ever since. At first, you were coughing up some colourless phlegm but the cough is now dry. You did have other cold symptoms but they have cleared up. You now have no symptoms other than the cough.

You have tried some over-the-counter remedies and hot drinks, but nothing has seemed to make it any better.

You cough at any time of day or night. It is not worse at any particular time. It is waking you up at night and so you are feeling tired during the day.

### Social history

Think about:
➤ marital status
➤ accommodation
➤ employment.

### Lifestyle

Think about:
➤ diet
➤ exercise
➤ smoking
➤ alcohol.

### Past medical history

You have had no serious illnesses or treatment in the past.

### Family history

You have no significant history of any illnesses in your family.

### Medication

You have been taking some cough sweets and linctus from the chemist.

### Allergies

None.

### Patient perspective

Consider your:
➤ temperament
➤ ideas about what is wrong
➤ concerns about what is wrong
➤ expectations of what you would like to happen next
➤ how you are likely to behave in the consultation
➤ how you are likely to respond to questions and discussion.

## SAMPLE BRIEF 7: TELEPHONE CONSULTATION

This scenario can be used to practise skills of negotiation on the telephone. The levels of challenge can be carefully set by the facilitator and simulated patient. This scenario can be further developed into a face-to-face encounter.

## Potential learning points

➤ **Medical** – the writing of letters/sick notes.
➤ **Psychological** – effects of anxiety on behaviour
➤ **Social** – appreciating the impact on the individual of complex social pressures
➤ **Communication** – practising the consultation skills needed to communicate with a patient on the telephone, negotiation and diffusing a potentially volatile situation
➤ **Teamwork** – exploring teamwork within a practice
➤ **Ethical** – issues of confidentiality.

## Simulated patient's brief

➤ Name: any
➤ Age range: working age
➤ Gender: any
➤ Ethnicity: any

## Setting of interaction

This consultation takes place in the reception area of the surgery.

## Reason for interaction

You have telephoned the doctor's surgery as your boss at work has asked you to provide a letter from the doctor to state that you were too ill to work 2 weeks ago.

## Background

You have been working for a small company for 4 months. Prior to this, you had been unemployed for several years. You are very anxious not to have time off work, as your employer looks very unfavourably on this.

Unfortunately, 2 weeks ago you suffered from a chest infection following a cold and you received antibiotics from the doctor. You were off work for a week, but your employer is insisting on a letter from the doctor to verify your illness, refusing to accept self-certification, as 'anyone could fill a form in when they felt like a few days off'.

You have called the surgery several times and even called in once to ask for this letter, but you have been fobbed off each time, and the letter has not materialised.

## Social history

You have lived alone since the death of your father 2 years ago. You had a brief relationship in your teens, but you have never had a serious relationship since. You hated school, and you left without any qualifications. Since then, you have found it very difficult to find and keep work. You are not sure why, but you never seem able to hold down a job.

## Lifestyle

You have smoked 20 cigarettes a day since you were in your late teens. You drink 3–4 pints when you go out, which varies according to how much money you have. You eat microwave meals and you don't like being preached to about how much fruit you should be eating. You do not take any formal exercise, although currently you cycle the 2 miles to work each day.

## Past medical history

You are an infrequent attender. Two weeks ago – antibiotics for chest infection.

## Family history

You have no significant family history.

## Medication

You take paracetamol when required, but no other medication.

### Allergies
You have no known allergies.

### Temperament
You are uneducated and under-confident, but you mask this by a very loud and brash manner, very quickly rising to anger.

### Ideas
You cannot see why the surgery cannot provide you with a letter, and you feel that they are not being straight with you, that they are trying to fob you off.

### Concerns
You are terrified that you may lose this job, and you are desperate that the receptionist sorts out this letter for you.

### Expectations
You are expecting that they will provide you with the letter this afternoon.

### Behaviour
You are determined that you will not be fobbed off this time, and you will state quite clearly that you will be calling into the surgery at 4 p.m. on your way to work and the letter had better be there. You can be rude and even quite threatening. You do not need to be reasonable or listen to reason.

If the practitioner shows empathy and concern, you may calm down, but you are determined that by the end of the day you will have your letter.

### Feelings
You are irritated that they don't seem to understand the seriousness of the situation, feeling that you are not asking for much – just a simple letter explaining why you were off work.

### Variations
The levels of emotion can be varied to present more or less challenge.

### Opening statement

'I need a letter for my boss.'

## Practitioner's brief
You work in a small general practice, with two doctors and a practice nurse. One of the doctors is away on annual leave until next week and the other has just left for a meeting. The practice nurse is on a training course this afternoon. You are alone on reception.

*Further developments if required*

If you check in the patient's file, there is no mention in the general practitiooner notes of the patient requiring a letter. Instead, you see that the patient was advised to self-certify on this occasion.

## Simulated patient's additional brief

It is 4 p.m. You are on your way to start your shift at 4.45 p.m. and you have called in as promised to collect your letter. You are calm at the moment, expecting the letter, but you have a naturally abrasive, rude manner. You are also anxious not to be late for your evening shift.

## Practitioner's additional brief

It is 4 p.m. Mr Barton comes into the surgery to collect his letter. The doctor has not yet returned from visits, following her meeting.

# Resources for role development

## BOOKS

*The Bell Jar* (1963), by Sylvia Plath
*The Comforts of Madness* (1988), by Paul Sayer
*The Curious Incident of the Dog in the Night-Time* (2003), by Mark Haddon
*My Left Foot* (1954), by Christy Brown
*One Flew Over the Cuckoo's Nest* (1962), by Ken Kesey

## FILMS

*A Beautiful Mind* (2001) directed by Ron Howard
*Children of a Lesser God* (1986) directed by Randa Haines
*The Hours* (2002) directed by Stephen Daldry
*I Am Sam* (2001) directed by Jesse Nelson
*Iris* (2001) directed by Richard Eyre
*Little Man Tate* (1991) directed by Jodie Foster
*The Madness of King George* (1994) directed by Nicholas Hytner
*The Notebook* (2004) directed by Nick Cassavetes
*Ordinary People* (1980) directed by Robert Redford
*Rain Man* (1988) directed by Barry Levinson
*What's Eating Gilbert Grape* (1993) directed by Lasse Hallström

# A list of mood indicators

The following are some physical indicators of emotional states and moods that you can use to help simulated patients develop their own way of conveying emotions clearly. It is helpful if the simulators are conscious of the messages given by certain physical movements; these movements can be more actively used when working with a struggling practitioner. There is a wide spectrum within each emotion and the simulated patients should be aware of the effects of each.

## DISTRESS AND SADNESS
➤ Looking down
➤ Swallowing
➤ Raising and furrowing the brow
➤ Twitching facial muscles, especially around the mouth
➤ Passing hands over face
➤ Wringing hands
➤ Staring at a fixed spot
➤ Crying (this should come as a result of feeling the character's emotions; however, if that is not happening, sometimes trying not to blink can make the eyes water).

## ANGER
➤ Pressing the lips together
➤ Making eye contact more intense
➤ Bringing the eyebrows together
➤ Becoming less talkative
➤ Making voice more determined
➤ Clenching fists and tensing muscles in body
➤ Speaking more slowly, as if in a controlled way
➤ Exaggerating hand movements
➤ Raising pitch of voice
➤ Raising volume of voice
➤ Lowering volume of voice.

## ANXIETY

➤ Speaking more rapidly
➤ Tense body posture
➤ Furrowing the brow
➤ Raising pitch of voice
➤ Raising volume of voice
➤ Looking around the room, upcast eyes
➤ Clipped speech
➤ Breathing rapidly and shallowly.

## FEAR

➤ Slowing pace
➤ Leaving silences
➤ Lowering pitch of voice
➤ Lowering volume of voice
➤ Looking around the room, downcast eyes
➤ Breathing rapidly and shallowly.

## SHOCK

➤ Silence
➤ Stillness
➤ Widening the eyes
➤ Furrowing the brow
➤ Breathing heavily.

## LYING

➤ Looking around the room before answering
➤ Hesitating before speaking
➤ After initial hesitation, speaking very quickly and confidently.

## RELUCTANCE TO DIVULGE INFORMATION

➤ Looking around the room before answering
➤ Hesitating before speaking
➤ Maintaining hesitation throughout a difficult topic of conversation.

This is not a comprehensive list but is intended to generate ideas. The main thing is to ask the simulated patients to be conscious of the non-verbal signs they are displaying that convey their emotional state.

# Communication skills

There are many models for organising a consultation and many aspects to teach practitioners. Obviously, you will need to know these in detail before teaching. The following outlines provide a concise overview of some of the more common consultation models; they also provide an idea of the level of detail that your simulated patients will find useful to have in order for them to understand the overall aims of teaching communication skills to practitioners.

## CALGARY-CAMBRIDGE GUIDE TO THE MEDICAL INTERVIEW
A standard consultation model.
- ➤ Initiating the session:
  - — preparation
  - — establishing initial rapport
  - — identifying the reason(s) for the consultation.
- ➤ Gathering information:
  - — exploration of the patient's problems to discover the:
    - • biomedical perspective
    - • patient's perspective
    - • background information, context.
- ➤ Physical examination.
- ➤ Explanation and planning:
  - — providing the correct type and amount of information
  - — aiding accurate recall and understanding
  - — achieving a shared understanding, incorporating the patient's illness framework
  - — planning shared decision-making.
- ➤ Closing the session:
  - — ensuring appropriate point of closure
  - — forward planning.

Throughout this process, the practitioner should also be focusing on:
➤ structure
 — making the organisation overt
 — attending to flow
➤ building the relationship
 — using appropriate non-verbal behaviour
 — developing rapport
 — involving the patient.

## NEIGHBOUR CONSULTATION MODEL

This is a five-stage model:
➤ Connecting: achieving a working rapport with the patient; getting on the same wavelength.
➤ Summarising: obtaining a sufficiently comprehensive idea of the patient's real reason for consulting you.
➤ Handing over: making sure the patient is happy with the outcome of the consultation.
➤ Safety-netting: planning for the unexpected.
➤ Housekeeping: taking care of yourself.

## HOSPITAL CLERKING CONSULTATION MODEL

Checklist:
➤ history of present complaint
➤ past medical history
➤ medication
➤ family history
➤ social history
➤ direct questions
➤ examination
➤ investigation
➤ diagnosis.

## BYRNE AND LONG CONSULTATION MODEL

There are six phases that form a logical structure to the consultation:
➤ The doctor establishes a relationship with the patient.
➤ The doctor either attempts to discover or actually discovers the reason for the patient's attendance.
➤ The doctor conducts a verbal or physical examination, or both.
➤ The doctor, or the doctor and the patient, or the patient (in that order of probability) considers the condition.
➤ The doctor and, occasionally, the patient detail treatment or further investigation.
➤ The consultation is terminated (the doctor usually does this).

## STOTT AND DAVIES CONSULTATION MODEL

This model has four parts:
- ➤ management of presenting problems
- ➤ modification of help-seeking behaviour
- ➤ management of continuing problems
- ➤ opportunistic health promotion.

## PENDLETON CONSULTATION MODEL

This model involves seven basic tasks:
- ➤ Define reason for attending:
  - — nature and history of problem
  - — aetiology
  - — patient's ideas, anxieties, expectations
  - — effects of the problem
- ➤ Consider other problems:
  - — continuing problems
  - — at-risk factors
- ➤ Doctor and patient choose an action for each problem
- ➤ Sharing understanding
- ➤ Involve patient in management, sharing appropriate responsibility
- ➤ Use time and resources appropriately
- ➤ Establish and maintain a positive relationship.

## STEWART AND ROTER CONSULTATION MODEL

This consultation model involves two frameworks.
- ➤ Patient presents problem
- ➤ Gathering information
- ➤ Parallel search of two frameworks:
  - — the patient's agenda
  - — the doctor's agenda
- ➤ Integration of two frameworks
- ➤ Explanation and planning.

# Six Hats Exercise – Edward de Bono

There are many techniques that can give structure to the discussion in a forum theatre situation. One commonly used one is Edward de Bono's Six Hats Exercise.

Here the observing participants would be divided into six groups and each group 'given' a hat to wear. They would then focus their observations using characteristics of their own particular hat.

The characteristics are as follows:

Green hat – this group would be creative and innovative in their view of the situation, exploring new ideas.

Yellow hat – this group would concentrate on the positive aspects of the situation and the behaviours demonstrated.

Black hat – this group would look at the potential dangers and threats, the difficult areas, the challenges.

White hat – this group would identify the hard facts inherent in the situation.

Red hat – this group would look at the emotional content within the interaction.

Blue hat – this group would look at the overall effects of the situation and try to bring all sides together.

The groups can swap hats at various points within the exercise in order to experience a different viewpoint.

# Suggested further reading

## WRITTEN RESOURCES

Barrows HS. Simulated patients in medical teaching. *Can Med Assoc J.* 1968; **98**(14): 674–6.

Barrows HS. *Simulated (Standardized) Patients and Other Human Simulations.* Chapel Hill, NC; Health Sciences Consortium; 1987.

Bingham L, Burrows PJ, Caird R, *et al.* Simulated surgery: a framework for the assessment of clinical competence. *Educ Gen Pract.* 1994; **5**: 143–50.

Bingham L, Burrows PJ, Caird R, *et al.* Simulated surgery: using standardized patients to assess clinical competence of GP registrars; a potential clinical component of the MRCGP examination. *Educ Gen Pract.* 1996; **7**: 102–11.

Byrne PS, Long BEL. *Doctors Talking to Patients.* London: RCGP Publications; 1976.

Callaway S, Bosshart DA, O'Donnell AA. Patient simulators in teaching patient education skills to family practice residents. *J Fam Pract.* 1977; **4**(4): 709–12.

Carroll JG, Schwartz MW, Ludwig S. An evaluation of simulated patients as instructors: implications for teaching medical interview skills. *J Med Educ.* 1981; **56**(6): 522–4.

Coll X, Papageorgiou A, Stanley A, Tarbuck A (eds) *Communication Skills in Mental Health Care: an introduction.* Oxford: Radcliffe Publishing; 2012.

Coonar AS, Dooley M, Daniels M, *et al.* The use of role-play in teaching medical students obstetrics and gynaecology. *Med Teach.* 1991; **13**(1): 49–53.

Corney R, editor. *Developing Communication and Counselling Skills in Medicine.* London: Tavistock/Routledge; 1991.

De Bono E. *Six Thinking Hats.* Toronto: Key Porter; 1985.

Fielding R. *Clinical Communication Skills.* Hong Kong: Hong Kong University Press; 1995.

Fraser RC. *Clinical Method: a general practice approach.* Oxford: Butterworth Heinemann; 1992.

General Medical Council. *Tomorrow's Doctors: recommendations on undergraduate medical education.* London: General Medical Council; 1993.

Hoppe RB, Farquhar LJ, Henry R, *et al.* Residents' attitudes towards and skills in counselling using undetected standardised patients. *J Gen Intern Med.* 1990; **5**(5): 415–20.

Johnstone K. *Improvisation and the Theatre*. London: Eyre Methuen; 1981.

Johnstone K. *Impro for Storytellers: theatresports and the art of making things happen* London: Faber and Faber; 1999.

Ker JS, Dowie A, Dowell J, *et al.* Twelve tips for maintaining a simulated patient bank. *Med Teach.* 2005; **27**(1): 4–9.

Koh KT, Goh LG, Tan T. Using role-play to teach consultation skills: the Singapore experience. *Med Teach.* 1991; **13**(1): 55–61.

Kurtz S, Silverman J, Benson J, *et al.* Marrying content and process in clinical method teaching: enhancing the Calcary-Cambridge guides. *Acad Med.* 2003; **78**(8): 802–9.

Kurtz S, Silverman J, Draper J. *Teaching and Learning Communication Skills in Medicine.* 2nd ed. Oxford: Radcliffe Publishing; 2005.

Laidlaw T, Kaufman DM, MacLeod H, *et al.* Relationship of communication skills assessment by experts, standardized patients and self-raters. *A presentation at the Association of Canadian Medical Colleges Annual Meeting.* 2004 Apr 24–27; Halifax, Nova Scotia.

Levenkron JC, Greenland P, Bowley M. Using patient instructors to teach behavioural counseling skills. *J Med Educ.* 1987; **62**(8): 665–72.

McAvoy BR. Teaching clinical skills to medical students: the use of simulated patients and videotaping in general practice. *Med Educ.* 1988; **22**(3): 193–9.

Maguire P. The use of patient simulation in training medical students in history-taking skills. *Med Biol Illus.* 1976; **26**(2): 91–5.

Maguire P, Roe P, Goldberg D, *et al.* The value of feedback in teaching interviewing skills to medical students. *Psychol Med.* 1978; **8**(4): 695–704.

Myerscough PR. *Talking with Patients: a basic clinical skill.* Oxford: Oxford University Press, Oxford; 1992.

Neighour RH. *The Inner Consultation.* Lancaster: MTP Press; 1987.

Nestel K, Muir E, Plant M, *et al.* Modelling the lay-expert for first year medical students: the actor-patient as teacher. *Med Teach.* 2002; **24**(5): 562–4.

Pendleton D, Schofield T, Tate P, *et al. The Consultation: an approach to teaching and learning.* Oxford: Oxford Medical Publications; 1984.

Pendleton D, Schofield T, Tate P, *et al. The New Consultation.* Oxford: Oxford University Press, Oxford; 2003.

Pololi LH. Standardised patients: as we evaluate so shall we reap. *Lancet.* 1995; **345**(8955): 966–8.

Quilligan S. Communication skills teaching: the challenge of giving effective feedback. *Clin Teach.* 2007; **4**(2): 100–5.

Sanson-Fisher RW, Poole AD. Simulated patients and the assessment of students' interpersonal skills. *Med Educ.* 1980; **14**(4): 249–53.

Sharp PC, Pearce KA, Konen JC, *et al.* Using standardized patient instructors to teach health promotion interviewing skills. *Fam Med.* 1996; **28**(2): 103–6.

Silverman J, Kurtz S, Draper J. The Calgary-Cambridge approach to communication skills teaching, 1: agenda-led outcome-based analysis of the consultation. *Educ Gen Pract.* 1996; **7**: 288–99.

Silverman J, Kurtz S, Draper J. The Calgary-Cambridge approach to communication skills teaching, 2: the Set-Go method of descriptive feedback. *Educ Gen Pract.* 1997; **8**: 16–23.

Silverman J, Kurtz S, Draper J. *Skills for Communicating with Patients.* 2nd ed. Oxford: Radcliffe Publishing; 2005.

Spencer J, Dales J. Meeting the needs of simulated patients and caring for the person behind them. *Med Educ.* 2006; **40**(1): 3–5.

Stanislavski C. *An Actor Prepares.* Hapgood ER, translator. New York, NY: Routledge; 1936.

Stewart M, Roter D, editors. *Communicating with Medical Patients.* Newbury Park, CA: Sage; 1989.

Stott NC, Davis RH. The exceptional potential in each primary care consultation. *J R Coll Gen Pract.* 1979; **29**(201): 201–5.

Tate P. *The Doctor's Communication Handbook.* 6th ed. Oxford: Radcliffe Publishing; 2010.

Thew R, Worrall P. The selection and training of patient-simulators for the assessment of consultation performance in simulated surgeries. *Educ Gen Pract.* 1998; **9**(2): 211–15.

Thistlethwaite J, Ridgeway G. *Making It Real: a practical guide to experiential learning of communication.* Oxford: Radcliffe Publishing; 2006.

Vu NV, Barrows H. Use of standardised patients in clinical assessments: recent developments and measurement findings. *Educ Res.* 1994; **23**(3): 23–30.

Wallace P. *Coaching Standardized Patients: for use in the assessment of clinical competence.* New York, NY: Springer; 2007.

Whitehouse C, Morris P, Marks B. The role of actors in teaching communication. *Med Educ.* 1984; **18**(4): 262–8.

## WEB-BASED RESOURCES
- www.skillscascade.com
- www.spots-online.co.uk
- http://en.wikipedia.org/wiki/Constantin_Stanislavski
- www.asme.org.uk
- www.aspih.com
- www.medschools.ac.uk

# Index

accessories 28–9
addiction 63
agencies, recruitment from 17, 21
aggression 28, 91, 101
allergies, in scenarios 64
anger 91, 166, 188–9, 191, 211

bad news scenarios 65, 91, 155
Barrows, Howard S 11–12
behaviours, effects of 44
bilingual scenarios 22, 49, 107–10, 192–6
body language
    definition of 181
    absence of 113–14
    and communication 92
    and emotions 28

cameos 20, 33, 112, 130
catering 75
characters
    behaviour of 65
    social circumstances of 25
    temperament and feelings of 64
    varying 31–2
clinical educators, associate 132
clinical skills
    in examinations, see examination
      stations, clinical skills
    teaching 126
clothing 28
co-facilitation 130
communication
    difficulties 110, 115, 118–19
    sensitive 159, 196
    in warm-ups 84
confidentiality 109, 153, 181
conflict, managing 6, 65–6, 155

consent 19, 99, 105, 153, 175, 182
consistency
    in examination sessions 53
    and opening statement 65–6
consultation skills, in examinations, see
    examination stations, consultation skills
consultation skills training
    benefits of 9–11
    cause and effect aspect 37
    practitioners' experience of 78
consultations, models of 213–15
cultural issues 22, 25, 50

depression 28, 63, 200
diabetes 124

emotional safety 155–6
emotions
    degrees of 91
    physical indicators of 211–12
    simulating 54, 59, 166
empathy
    definition of 182
    in feedback 149
ethical issues, in scenarios 62
ethnicity, in scenarios 62
examination candidates, simulating 59
examination/recruitment preparation
    sessions 172–6
examination sessions
    core competencies for 21–2
    marking criteria for 58
    scenarios for 54, 60, 67
    training for 52–8
    variations in process 59
examination stations
    clinical skills 165

Printed and bound by CPI Group (UK) Ltd, Croydon, CR0 4YY

23/10/2024

01777678-0008